Filipino Recipes
Made Meatless

A PHILIPPINE VEGETARIAN COOKBOOK

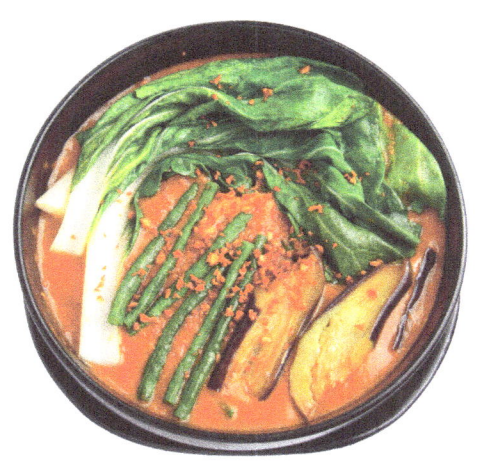

Janine Reyes, USRN

DISCLAIMER

Table of CONTENTS
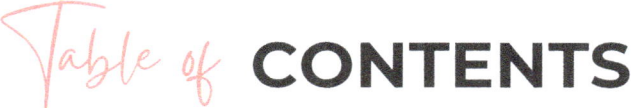

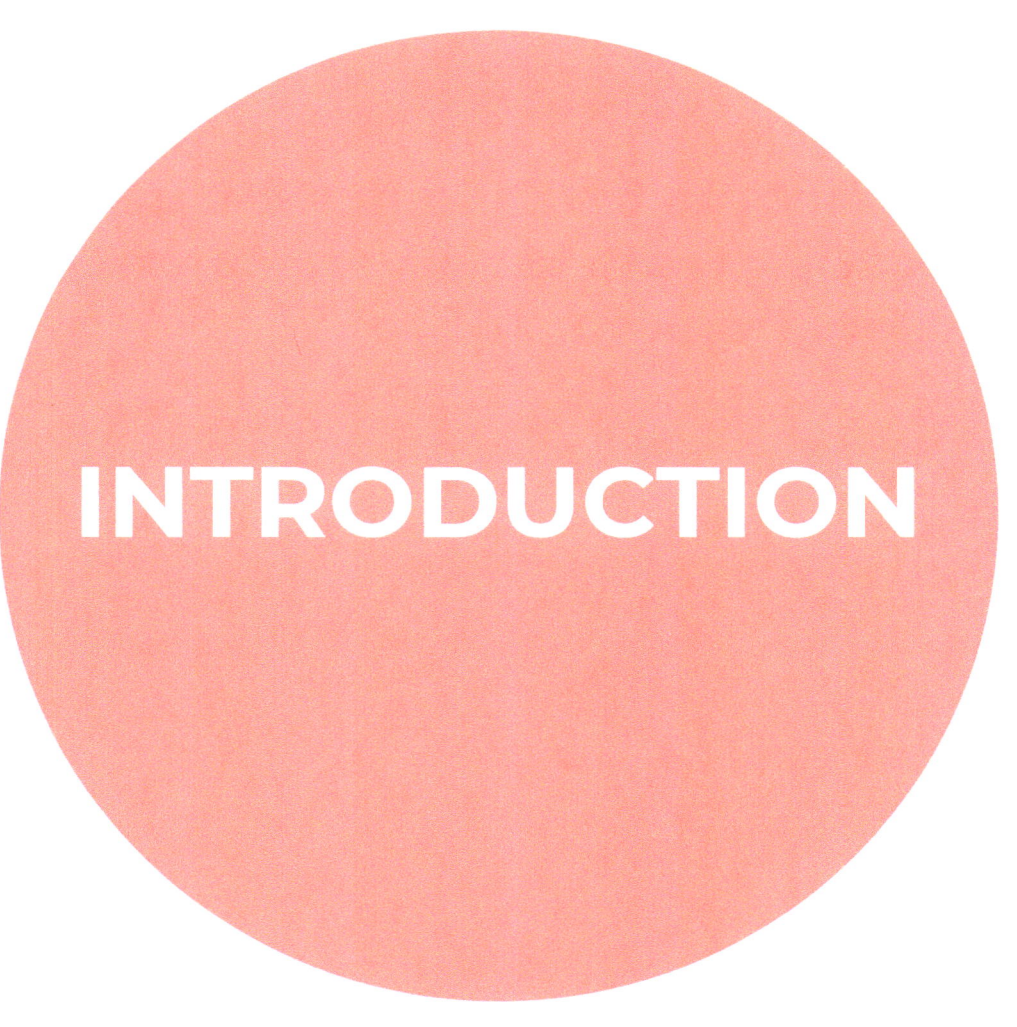

INTRODUCTION

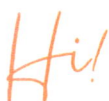

Welcome to "Filipino Recipes Made Meatless: A Vegetarian Cookbook for All"!

This cookbook is a celebration of the rich and vibrant flavors of Filipino cuisine, reimagined through a vegetarian lens. Here, you will discover authentic recipes that honor the traditions of my homeland while embracing a plant-based lifestyle. Whether you are a lifelong vegetarian, someone exploring new dietary choices, or simply a fan of Filipino food, this book offers something for everyone. Each recipe is designed to bring the warmth and joy of Filipino cooking into your kitchen, encouraging you to share these delightful dishes with family and friends.

My Journey in creating this cookbook

My name is Janine Reyes, and I am a proud Filipino-American nurse and mother, dedicated to sharing the flavors and traditions of my culture through cooking. Born in the Philippines and immigrating to the United States at the age of six, my journey has been one of embracing my heritage while adapting to a new environment. Growing up, my kitchen was filled with the vibrant aromas of Filipino dishes, lovingly prepared by my mother and grandmother. These meals were more than just nourishment; they were a way to connect with family, celebrate special occasions, and honor our cultural roots.

As a mother of two beautiful daughters, Katie and Lovella, I am passionate about instilling a love for our culinary heritage in them. My commitment to healthy living led me to explore vegetarian cooking, and I found joy in transforming traditional recipes into plant-based versions. This journey has allowed me to create new memories while honoring the flavors of my childhood.

HOW TO BEST USE THIS *Cookbook*

This cookbook is structured to guide you through the essentials of Filipino vegetarian cooking. Here's how to make the most of it:

1. **Understanding Filipino Vegetarian Cuisine:** Begin by exploring the essence of Filipino flavors and the benefits of a vegetarian diet. This section will help you appreciate the ingredients you'll be using and the cultural significance behind them.

2. **Filipino Cooking Essentials:** Familiarize yourself with key ingredients, common cooking techniques, and tips for adapting traditional recipes into vegetarian versions. This knowledge will empower you to experiment and create your own culinary masterpieces.

3. **Delicious Recipes:** Dive into a variety of recipes, organized by categories such as appetizers, main dishes, soups, and desserts. Each recipe includes preparation and cooking times, serving sizes, and nutritional information to help you plan your meals.

4. **Meal Planning Made Easy:** Discover quick meal prep tips and guidance on creating your own Filipino vegetarian meal plans, making it easier to incorporate these delicious dishes into your everyday life.

5. **Cultural Context and Personal Stories:** Enjoy personal anecdotes and stories that highlight the role of food in Filipino culture, connecting you deeper to this rich culinary heritage.

I invite you to embark on this flavorful journey with me. Let's celebrate the beauty of Filipino cuisine while embracing a vegetarian lifestyle. Together, we can create lasting memories around the dinner table, one delicious dish at a time.

Understanding
FILIPINO
VEGETARIAN
CUISINE

THE ESSENCE OF FILIPINO FLAVORS

Welcome to the delightful world of Filipino flavors! If you've ever indulged in a Filipino meal, you know that our cuisine is a beautiful symphony of tastes, each note carefully crafted from our rich history and diverse culture. The key to these vibrant flavors lies in a few beloved elements that come together to create dishes that are not just food but a celebration of life.

- **Sourness:** Ah, the unmistakable tang of **sinigang** or the zesty punch of **calamansi**! Sourness is a cornerstone of Filipino cooking, bringing a bright and refreshing contrast to many dishes. Whether it's the bold flavor of tamarind in a sour soup or the tartness of green mangoes in a salad, this sour note awakens the palate and makes every bite a little more exciting.

- **Umami:** This savory depth is what makes our dishes so comforting and satisfying. In traditional recipes, umami often comes from fish sauce or shrimp paste, but in our vegetarian adaptations, we can find that savory richness in mushrooms, soy sauce, and even roasted vegetables. It's all about layering flavors to achieve that delicious complexity.

- **Aromatics:** The intoxicating scents of garlic, onions, and ginger sizzling in a pan can transport you back to your childhood kitchen. These aromatics are the heartbeat of Filipino cooking, creating a warm and inviting atmosphere as they fill your home with their comforting fragrance.

- **Herbs and Spices:** Fresh herbs like **cilantro** and **green onions** add that final flourish to our meals, while spices like black pepper and chili infuse heat and brightness. They bring life to every dish, creating a beautiful balance that's quintessentially Filipino.

By diving into these elements, you'll discover how traditional Filipino dishes can be reimagined as vegetarian delights without losing that beloved essence.

Benefits of a **VEGETARIAN DIET**

Now, let's talk about the wonderful benefits of adopting a vegetarian lifestyle. Making this choice can positively impact your health, the environment, and even your soul!

(01) HEALTH BENEFITS

A vegetarian diet is often packed with vibrant fruits, crunchy vegetables, whole grains, and wholesome nuts and seeds. Not only does this mean you're nourishing your body with essential nutrients, but studies have shown that a plant-based diet can lower the risk of chronic diseases. Plus, it can help you feel more energized and vibrant—who doesn't want that?

(02) ENVIRONMENTAL IMPACT

Our planet is in need of a little TLC, and choosing vegetarian options is one way to contribute to its well-being. Plant-based foods generally have a lower carbon footprint compared to meat, which means fewer greenhouse gases and less water usage. Your choices at the dinner table can help create a healthier Earth for future generations.

(03) ETHICAL CONSIDERATIONS

For many, the decision to go vegetarian stems from a deep compassion for animals. Embracing a vegetarian lifestyle reflects a commitment to kindness and respect for all living beings, aligning your values with your food choices.

Embracing Plant-Based Cooking
IN FILIPINO CULTURE

In Filipino culture, food is about more than just sustenance; it's a way to connect, celebrate, and create lasting memories with loved ones. As we embrace vegetarian cooking, we're not just adapting recipes—we're continuing a rich culinary tradition.

01 INNOVATIVE RECIPES

The beauty of Filipino cuisine is its adaptability. Traditional favorites like **Kare-Kare** or **Adobo** can be transformed into delicious vegetarian versions without sacrificing the flavors we love. Think of it as a culinary adventure—experimenting with new ingredients and techniques while honoring our roots.

02 COMMUNITY AND SHARING

Food brings us together. When you prepare and share vegetarian dishes, you're not just feeding your loved ones; you're creating moments of joy and connection. There's something magical about gathering around the table, sharing stories, and enjoying the fruits of your labor together.

03 CULTURAL PRESERVATION

By reinventing traditional recipes as vegetarian delights, we're preserving our culinary heritage for future generations. It's a way to honor our past while embracing the present and future, ensuring that the flavors of our culture continue to thrive.

As you explore the world of Filipino vegetarian cuisine, remember that food is a reflection of love, culture, and community. Each recipe in this book is a piece of my heart, crafted with the hope that it brings warmth and joy to your table. Let's celebrate our heritage together, one delicious bite at a time!

FILIPINO COOKING ESSENTIALS

Key Ingredients FOR FILIPINO VEGETARIAN COOKING

As we embark on this flavorful journey through Filipino vegetarian cooking, it's essential to familiarize ourselves with the key ingredients that will bring our dishes to life. Here are some staples that you'll find in many Filipino kitchens, perfect for creating delicious plant-based meals:

Rice: The heart of Filipino meals, rice is a staple that accompanies nearly every dish. Whether it's steamed jasmine rice or fragrant coconut rice, this versatile grain serves as the perfect base for your meals.

Coconut Milk: A beloved ingredient in Filipino cuisine, coconut milk adds creaminess and richness to dishes like **Kare-Kare** and **Ginataang** (cooked in coconut milk). It's also a key component in desserts like **Bibingka** and **Leche Flan**.

Soy Sauce: This umami-rich condiment is used in marinades, stir-fries, and soups. It adds depth of flavor to dishes and is an excellent substitute for fish sauce in vegetarian recipes.

Tamarind: Known for its tangy flavor, tamarind is often used in sour dishes like **Sinigang**. You can find tamarind paste or fresh tamarind in Asian markets, making it easy to incorporate that signature sourness into your meals.

Miso Paste: A fermented soybean product, miso adds a savory depth to soups and marinades. It's a fantastic way to enhance the umami flavor in vegetarian dishes.

Fresh Vegetables: A colorful array of vegetables is essential in Filipino cooking. Common choices include eggplant, green beans, bitter melon, and leafy greens like **kangkong** (water spinach) or **pechay** (bok choy). Fresh herbs like cilantro and green onions also bring brightness to your dishes.

Chili Peppers: For those who enjoy a kick of heat, chili peppers are often included in Filipino recipes. From mild to spicy, they add flavor and excitement to your meals.

COMMON COOKING TECHNIQUES AND TERMS

Understanding the cooking techniques and terms used in Filipino cuisine will empower you to recreate these dishes with confidence. Here are some essential techniques to get you started:

 ### SAUTÉING (SAUTÉ)

This technique involves cooking ingredients in oil over medium heat until they are soft and fragrant. It's the foundation for many Filipino dishes, starting with the holy trinity of garlic, onion, and ginger.

 ### SIMMERING (SINIGANG)

Simmering is a gentle cooking method that allows flavors to meld while keeping ingredients tender. It's commonly used in soups and stews, such as **Sinigang**, where the ingredients are cooked in a broth until they're perfectly tender.

 ### STEAMING (STEAM)

Steaming is a healthy cooking method often used for vegetables and rice cakes like **puto** (steamed rice cakes). It preserves the nutrients and vibrant colors of the ingredients.

 ### BRAISING (BRAISE)

This technique involves cooking ingredients slowly in a small amount of liquid. It's often used for meats, but you can easily apply it to hearty vegetables and legumes for deep flavor.

 ### ROASTING (ROAST)

Roasting enhances the natural sweetness of vegetables and adds a delicious caramelized flavor. It's perfect for preparing vegetables like eggplant and squash.

TIPS FOR ADAPTING TRADITIONAL RECIPES TO VEGETARIAN VERSIONS

Transforming traditional Filipino recipes into vegetarian delights is a rewarding and creative process. Here are some tips to help you make those adaptations successfully:

1. **Identify the Key Flavors:** When adapting a recipe, focus on the primary flavors and textures. For example, in **Adobo**, the savory and tangy notes can be maintained by using mushrooms or tofu in place of meat.

2. **Use Plant-Based Proteins:** Experiment with tofu, tempeh, seitan, or legumes like chickpeas and lentils to replace meat in recipes. These ingredients can absorb flavors beautifully and provide the heartiness that many Filipino dishes require.

3. **Enhance Umami:** Incorporate ingredients that provide umami, such as mushrooms, soy sauce, miso paste, or nutritional yeast. These will help achieve the depth of flavor that is characteristic of traditional Filipino dishes.

4. **Adjust Cooking Times:** Keep in mind that plant-based proteins may require different cooking times than meat. Be sure to monitor the texture and doneness of your ingredients to ensure they're cooked perfectly.

5. **Don't Forget the Seasonings:** Filipino cuisine relies heavily on aromatic seasonings and spices. Be generous with garlic, ginger, and herbs to create that comforting and familiar flavor profile.

6. **Have Fun and Experiment:** Cooking is an art, and adapting recipes is a chance to get creative. Don't be afraid to try new ingredients or techniques to make each dish your own!

With these essentials in your culinary toolbox, you're ready to dive into the world of Filipino vegetarian cooking. Each recipe in this book is an opportunity to explore, experiment, and enjoy the rich flavors of our beloved cuisine while honoring a plant-based lifestyle.

APPETIZERS AND SNACKS

Vegetarian Lumpiang Shanghai

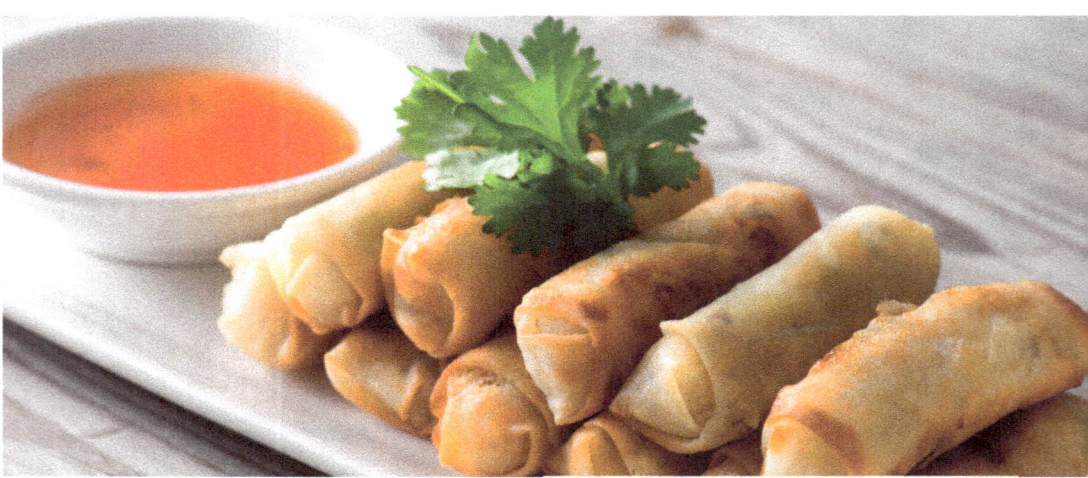

Vegetarian Lumpiang Shanghai is a delightful twist on the classic Filipino spring rolls, filled with a savory combination of vegetables and tofu, wrapped in a crispy shell. This dish is often a staple during celebrations and gatherings, evoking memories of family feasts and joyous occasions in the Philippines.

Author's Personal Connection

As a child, I remember my grandmother meticulously preparing Lumpiang Shanghai during family gatherings. The aroma of garlic and sautéed vegetables would fill the kitchen, drawing everyone together. Each roll was a work of love, and everyone eagerly awaited their turn to enjoy these crispy delights. Now, as I pass down this recipe to my daughters, I hope to create those same cherished memories and instill in them our rich culinary heritage.

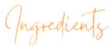
Ingredients

For the Filling:
- 1 cup firm tofu, crumbled
- 1 cup carrots, finely chopped
- 1 cup green beans, finely chopped
- 1 cup cabbage, shredded
- 1/2 cup onions, finely chopped
- 3 cloves garlic, minced
- 2 tablespoons soy sauce
- 1 tablespoon oyster sauce (vegetarian version)
- 1 teaspoon salt
- 1/2 teaspoon black pepper
- 1 tablespoon cooking oil

For the Wrapping:
- 20-25 spring roll wrappers
- Oil for frying

Servings:	4-6
Preparation Time:	30 min.
Cooking Time:	15 min.
Total Time:	45 min.

Nutrition:

Calories	180
Protein	8 g
Fat	9 g
Carbohydrates	20 g
Fiber	3 g
Sodium	300 mg

Instructions

Prepare the Filling
- In a large pan, heat the cooking oil over medium heat. Sauté the garlic and onions until fragrant.
- Add the crumbled tofu and cook until slightly browned.
- Stir in the carrots, green beans, and cabbage. Cook for about 5-7 minutes until the vegetables are tender.
- Add the soy sauce, oyster sauce, salt, and pepper. Mix well and remove from heat. Allow the filling to cool.

Assemble the Spring Rolls
- Lay a spring roll wrapper on a clean surface, with one corner pointing towards you.
- Spoon about 2 tablespoons of the filling onto the wrapper, forming a log shape.
- Fold the bottom corner over the filling, then fold in the sides. Roll tightly towards the top corner, sealing the edge with a bit of water.

Fry the Spring Rolls
- In a deep pan, heat oil over medium-high heat. Once hot, carefully add the spring rolls in batches, frying until golden brown and crispy (about 3-4 minutes).
- Remove and drain on paper towels.

Serve
- Serve hot with sweet and sour sauce or vinegar dipping sauce.

Kwek-Kwek

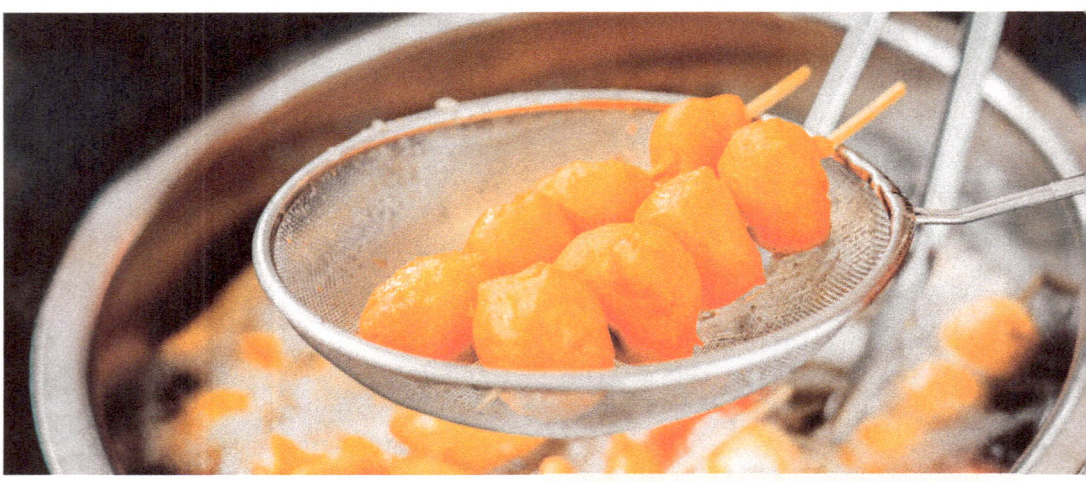

Kwek-Kwek is a beloved Filipino street food that features quail eggs coated in a bright orange batter and deep-fried until crispy. This vegetarian adaptation uses plant-based ingredients to create a similar taste and texture, allowing everyone to enjoy this iconic snack without compromising dietary choices.

Author's Personal Connection

Growing up, Kwek-Kwek was a favorite treat during family outings and festivals. I remember the excitement of watching street vendors prepare these golden, crunchy delights, the smell of frying batter wafting through the air as we eagerly awaited our turn. Now, I enjoy making a vegetarian version for my daughters, sharing the joy of this beloved snack and the vibrant street food culture of the Philippines.

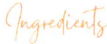
Ingredients

For the Plant-Based "Eggs"
- 1 cup chickpeas (cooked and mashed)
- 1/4 cup nutritional yeast
- 1 tablespoon cornstarch
- 1/2 teaspoon turmeric powder (for color)
- 1/2 teaspoon garlic powder
- Salt and pepper to taste
- 1/4 cup water (as needed)

For the Batter
- 1 cup all-purpose flour
- 1/2 cup cornstarch
- 1 teaspoon baking powder
- 1 teaspoon paprika
- 1 teaspoon salt
- 1 cup water (adjust for batter consistency)
- 1 tablespoon vegetable oil

For Frying
- Oil for deep frying

Servings:	**4**
Preparation Time:	**20 min.**
Cooking Time:	**15 min.**
Total Time:	**35 min.**

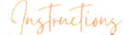
Nutrition:

Calories	**220**
Protein	**10 g**
Fat	**12 g**
Carbohydrates	**24 g**
Fiber	**4 g**
Sodium	**400 mg**

Instructions

Prepare the Plant-Based "Eggs"
- In a bowl, combine the mashed chickpeas, nutritional yeast, cornstarch, turmeric, garlic powder, salt, and pepper. Mix well.
- Gradually add water until the mixture holds together but is not too wet. Form into small balls (about the size of quail eggs) and set aside.

Make the Batter
- In another bowl, whisk together the flour, cornstarch, baking powder, paprika, and salt.
- Gradually add water and vegetable oil, mixing until you achieve a smooth batter. It should be thick enough to coat the chickpea balls.

Heat the Oil
- In a deep pan or pot, heat oil over medium-high heat for frying. Ensure the oil is hot enough by dropping a small amount of batter into it; if it sizzles, it's ready.

Coat and Fry the "Eggs"
- Dip each chickpea ball into the batter, allowing excess to drip off. Carefully place them into the hot oil.
- Fry until golden brown and crispy, about 3-4 minutes. Fry in batches to avoid overcrowding.

Drain and Serve
- Remove from oil and drain on paper towels. Serve hot with a vinegar dipping sauce or sweet and spicy sauce.

Vegetable Pancit Canton

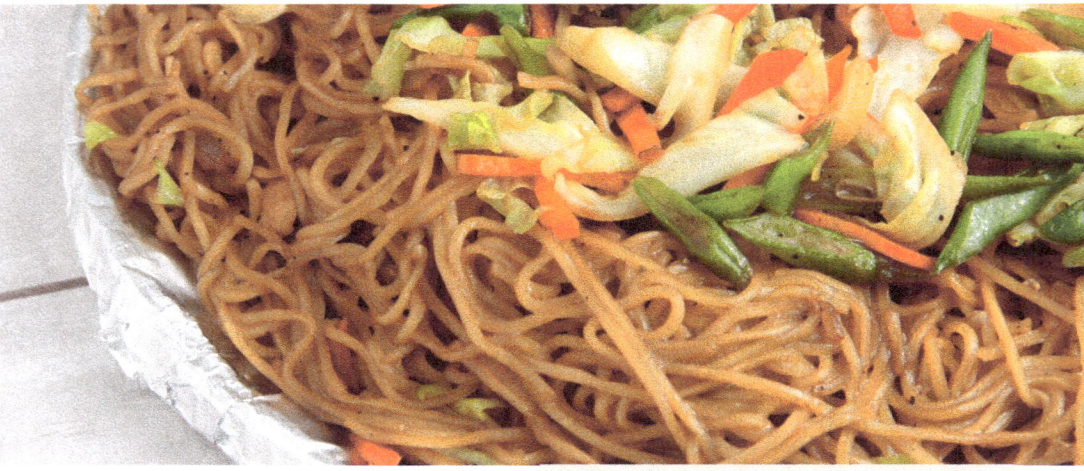

Vegetable Pancit Canton is a vibrant stir-fried noodle dish that showcases a medley of fresh vegetables tossed with chewy egg noodles. Traditionally served during celebrations and family gatherings, this vegetarian version captures the essence of Filipino cuisine while being a wholesome and satisfying meal.

Author's Personal Connection

Growing up, Pancit Canton was a staple at family gatherings and birthday celebrations. I fondly remember my mother preparing this dish, ensuring it was loaded with vibrant vegetables and savory flavors. The joy of sharing a big platter of Pancit with family and friends around the table is a cherished memory I love to recreate with my daughters, teaching them the importance of food in our culture and the joy of sharing.

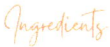

Ingredients

For the Noodles
- 12 ounces Pancit Canton noodles (egg noodles, can substitute with wheat noodles for a vegan option)

For the Stir-Fry
- 2 tablespoons vegetable oil
- 1 medium onion, sliced
- 3 cloves garlic, minced
- 1 cup carrots, julienned
- 1 cup bell peppers (red and green), sliced
- 1 cup snow peas or green beans, trimmed
- 1 cup cabbage, shredded
- 1/2 cup shiitake mushrooms, sliced (or any preferred mushroom)

For the Sauce
- 3 tablespoons soy sauce
- 1 tablespoon oyster sauce (vegetarian version)
- 1 tablespoon sesame oil
- 1/2 teaspoon black pepper
- Salt to taste

Servings:	4-6
Preparation Time:	15 min.
Cooking Time:	15 min.
Total Time:	30 min.

Nutrition:

Calories	280
Protein	8 g
Fat	10 g
Carbohydrates	42 g
Fiber	4 g
Sodium	600 mg

Instructions

Cook the Noodles
- In a large pot of boiling water, cook the Pancit Canton noodles according to package instructions until al dente. Drain and set aside. Toss with a little oil to prevent sticking.

Stir-Fry the Vegetables
- In a large skillet or wok, heat the vegetable oil over medium heat. Add the sliced onions and minced garlic, sautéing until fragrant.
- Add the carrots and bell peppers, cooking for about 2-3 minutes.
- Stir in the snow peas or green beans and cabbage, cooking until just tender, about 2-3 minutes.
- Add the sliced mushrooms and cook for an additional 2 minutes.

Combine Noodles and Sauce
- Add the cooked noodles to the skillet with the vegetables. Pour in the soy sauce, oyster sauce, sesame oil, black pepper, and salt. Toss everything together until the noodles are well coated and heated through.

Serve
- Transfer the Vegetable Pancit Canton to a serving platter. Garnish with chopped green onions or fried garlic if desired. Serve hot.

Chicharrón

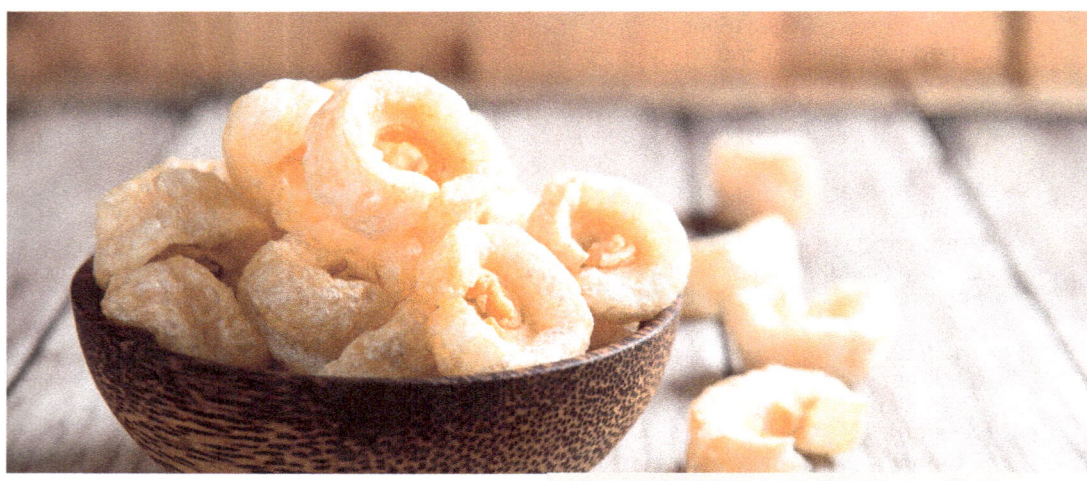

Vegetarian Chicharrón is a crispy, savory snack that replaces traditional pork rinds with crunchy tofu skins. This delightful treat is perfect for sharing and can be enjoyed as an appetizer or a topping for various dishes. It brings the same satisfying crunch and flavor to the table while keeping it plant-based.

Author's Personal Connection

Chicharrón has always held a special place in my heart. I remember the excitement of visiting local markets in the Philippines, where vendors would showcase their crispy pork rinds, and the aroma would draw us in. Sharing this crunchy delight with family during special occasions made it a favorite treat. Now, I love making this vegetarian version for my daughters, allowing them to enjoy the same crispy indulgence while embracing our culinary heritage.

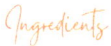
Ingredients

For the Tofu Skins
- 8 ounces crispy tofu skins (also known as tofu puffs or bean curd sheets)

For the Marinade
- 2 tablespoons soy sauce
- 1 tablespoon rice vinegar
- 1 teaspoon garlic powder
- 1 teaspoon onion powder
- 1/2 teaspoon paprika
- Salt and pepper to taste

For Frying
- Oil for deep frying

Servings:	4
Preparation Time:	15 min.
Cooking Time:	10 min.
Total Time:	25 min.

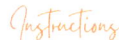
Nutrition:

Calories	150
Protein	10 g
Fat	8 g
Carbohydrates	10 g
Fiber	1 g
Sodium	400 mg

Instructions

Prepare the Tofu Skins
- If using dried tofu skins, soak them in warm water for about 30 minutes until pliable. Drain and pat dry. If using fresh crispy tofu skins, cut them into bite-sized pieces.

Marinate the Tofu Skins
- In a bowl, combine the soy sauce, rice vinegar, garlic powder, onion powder, paprika, salt, and pepper. Add the tofu skins and gently toss to coat. Let them marinate for 10-15 minutes.

Heat the Oil
- In a deep pan or pot, heat oil over medium-high heat. Ensure the oil is hot enough by dropping a small piece of tofu skin into it; if it sizzles, it's ready.

Fry the Tofu Skins
- Carefully add the marinated tofu skins to the hot oil in batches. Fry until golden brown and crispy, about 3-5 minutes. Avoid overcrowding the pan to ensure even cooking.

Drain and Serve
- Remove the crispy tofu skins from the oil and drain on paper towels. Serve hot, with a side of vinegar or spicy dipping sauce for extra flavor.

MAIN DISHES

Adobong Sitaw

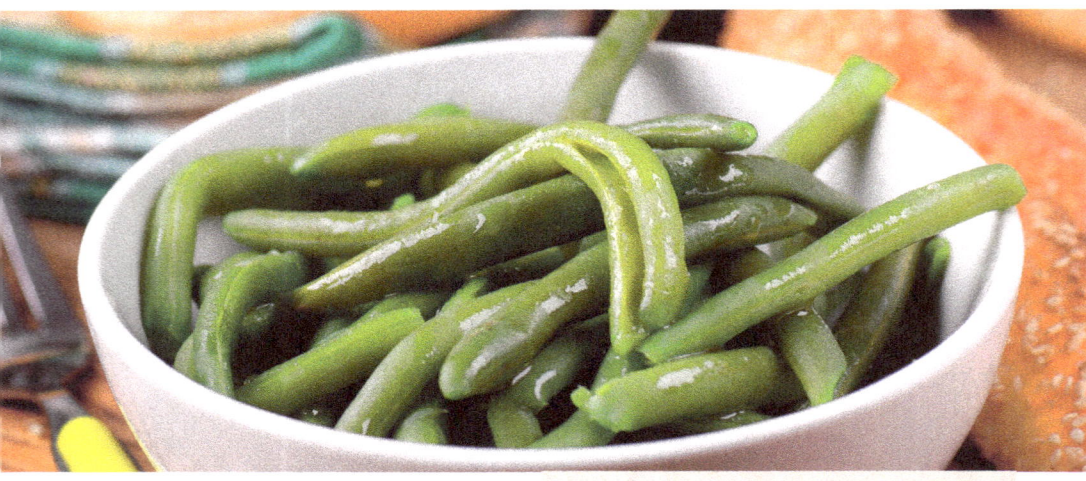

Adobong Sitaw is a delightful Filipino dish where tender string beans are simmered in a rich blend of soy sauce, vinegar, garlic, and spices. This vegetarian adaptation captures the essence of traditional adobo while highlighting the crispness of the string beans, making it a perfect side dish or main course served with rice.

Author's Personal Connection

Adobong Sitaw was a regular dish at our family table, often prepared by my mother with fresh vegetables from our garden. I have fond memories of helping her snap the string beans and watching as they transformed into a flavorful adobo. Now, I cherish the opportunity to pass this recipe to my daughters, sharing the story of our family's love for cooking and the importance of using fresh ingredients.

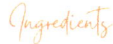
Ingredients

For the Adobo
- 1 pound string beans (sitaw), trimmed and cut into 2-inch pieces
- 2 tablespoons vegetable oil
- 1 medium onion, sliced
- 4 cloves garlic, minced
- 1/4 cup soy sauce
- 1/4 cup white vinegar
- 1 teaspoon black pepper
- 1 bay leaf
- 1/2 cup water
- Salt to taste

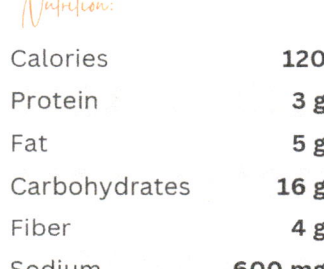

Servings:	4
Preparation Time:	10 min.
Cooking Time:	20 min.
Total Time:	30 min.

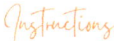
Nutrition:

Calories	120
Protein	3 g
Fat	5 g
Carbohydrates	16 g
Fiber	4 g
Sodium	600 mg

Instructions

Sauté the Aromatics
- In a large skillet or pot, heat the vegetable oil over medium heat. Add the sliced onions and minced garlic, sautéing until fragrant and the onions become translucent.

Add the String Beans
- Stir in the string beans and cook for about 2-3 minutes until they start to soften.

Make the Adobo Sauce
- Add the soy sauce, vinegar, black pepper, bay leaf, and water to the skillet. Stir to combine all the ingredients.

Simmer
- Bring the mixture to a simmer. Cover the pot and let it cook for about 10-15 minutes, or until the string beans are tender but still crisp. Stir occasionally and adjust seasoning with salt if needed.

Serve
- Remove the bay leaf before serving. Serve hot over steamed rice.

Pinakbet

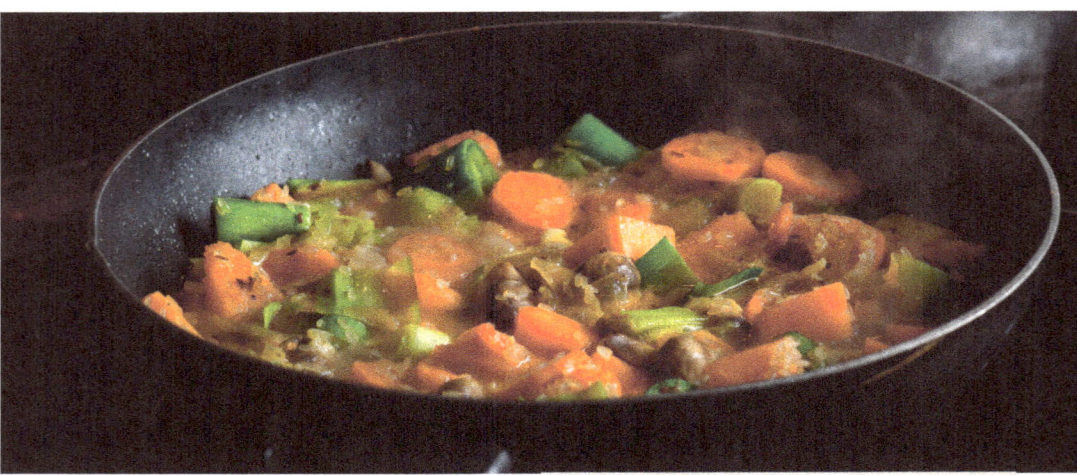

Pinakbet is a hearty and flavorful vegetable stew from the Philippines, traditionally made with a variety of vegetables and flavored with shrimp paste. This vegetarian version replaces the shrimp paste with a combination of spices and seasonings, allowing the natural sweetness of the vegetables to shine through. It's a nourishing dish that's both comforting and satisfying, perfect for any meal.

Author's Personal Connection

Growing up, Pinakbet was a staple in our household, especially during harvest season when our garden was overflowing with fresh vegetables. My mother would prepare this dish with whatever was in season, teaching me the importance of using local produce. Now, I love making this vegetarian version for my daughters, sharing the vibrant flavors and the story of our family's connection to the land and its bounty.

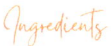
Ingredients

For the Stew
- 1 tablespoon vegetable oil
- 1 medium onion, sliced
- 4 cloves garlic, minced
- 1 medium tomato, chopped
- 1 cup eggplant, sliced into rounds
- 1 cup zucchini or pattypan squash, sliced
- 1 cup bitter melon (ampalaya), sliced (optional)
- 1 cup okra, trimmed
- 1 cup string beans (sitaw), cut into 2-inch pieces
- 1 cup squash (kabocha or butternut), cubed
- 1/4 cup water or vegetable broth
- 2 tablespoons soy sauce
- 1 tablespoon miso paste (for umami flavor)
- Salt and pepper, to taste
- Fresh basil or bitter melon leaves for garnish (optional)

Servings:	4-6
Preparation Time:	15 min.
Cooking Time:	30 min.
Total Time:	45 min.

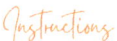
Nutrition:

Calories	150
Protein	5 g
Fat	4 g
Carbohydrates	25 g
Fiber	6 g
Sodium	500 mg

Instructions

Sauté Aromatics
- In a large pot or deep skillet, heat the vegetable oil over medium heat. Add the sliced onions and minced garlic, sautéing until fragrant and the onions are translucent.

Add Tomatoes
- Stir in the chopped tomatoes and cook until they soften and release their juices, about 3-4 minutes.

Add the Vegetables
- Add the eggplant, zucchini, bitter melon (if using), okra, string beans, and squash to the pot. Stir well to combine.

Season the Stew
- Pour in the water or vegetable broth, soy sauce, and miso paste. Mix well and bring the mixture to a gentle simmer. Cover the pot and let it cook for about 15-20 minutes, or until the vegetables are tender but still vibrant.

Adjust Seasoning
- Taste and adjust seasoning with salt and pepper as needed. If you prefer a stronger flavor, add more soy sauce or a bit of vegetable broth.

Serve
- Garnish with fresh basil or bitter melon leaves if desired. Serve hot with steamed rice.

Sinigang na baboy

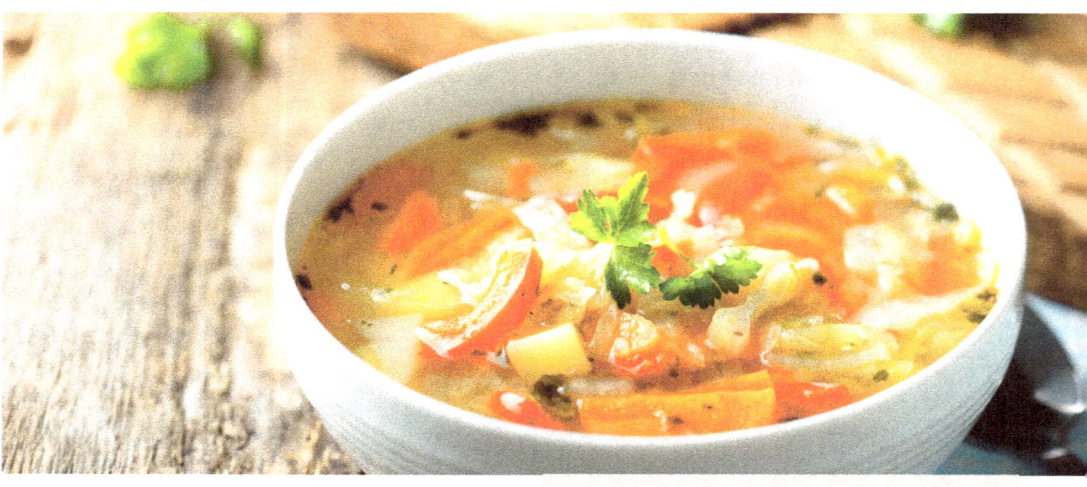

Sinigang is a traditional Filipino sour soup known for its tangy flavor, typically achieved through tamarind or other souring agents. This vegetarian version features a medley of fresh vegetables like radish, eggplant, and leafy greens, simmered in a flavorful broth that embodies the comforting and vibrant essence of Filipino cuisine.

Author's Personal Connection

Sinigang na Baboy has always been a family favorite in our home. I remember my mother preparing this dish on rainy days, filling the house with its inviting aroma. The sourness of the soup would warm our hearts and bring us all together around the table. Now, as I cook this vegetarian version for my daughters, I hope to share the same comfort and love that my family experienced with this iconic dish.

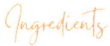
Ingredients

For the Broth
- 1 tablespoon vegetable oil
- 1 medium onion, quartered
- 4 cloves garlic, minced
- 1 medium tomato, quartered
- 1 radish (labanos), sliced
- 1 cup eggplant, sliced
- 1 cup green beans (sitaw), trimmed
- 1 cup water spinach (kangkong) or spinach
- 1 cup water
- 1/2 cup tamarind paste or 1-2 cups fresh tamarind (or use a souring agent like calamansi or green mango)
- 2 tablespoons soy sauce
- 1 teaspoon salt (or to taste)
- 1/2 teaspoon black pepper
- 1-2 green chili peppers (optional, for heat)

Servings:	**4-6**
Preparation Time:	**15 min.**
Cooking Time:	**30 min.**
Total Time:	**45 min.**

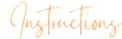
Nutrition:

Calories	**120**
Protein	**4 g**
Fat	**3 g**
Carbohydrates	**20 g**
Fiber	**5 g**
Sodium	**600 mg**

Instructions

Sauté the Aromatics
- In a large pot, heat the vegetable oil over medium heat. Add the quartered onions and minced garlic, sautéing until fragrant and the onions become translucent.

Add the Tomatoes
- Stir in the quartered tomatoes and cook until they soften, about 3-4 minutes.

Prepare the Broth
- Add the sliced radish, eggplant, and green beans to the pot. Pour in the water and bring to a boil. Reduce the heat and let it simmer for about 10 minutes until the vegetables begin to soften.

Add the Tamarind
- If using fresh tamarind, boil it in a separate pot with a little water until soft, then mash and strain the juice into the soup. If using tamarind paste, simply add it to the pot and stir well. Adjust the sourness to your preference by adding more tamarind or souring agent.

Season and Finish
- Add the soy sauce, salt, black pepper, and green chili peppers (if using). Stir in the water spinach (kangkong) or spinach and cook for an additional 2-3 minutes until the greens are wilted.

Serve
- Taste and adjust the seasoning as needed. Serve hot over steamed rice.

Tinolang Manok

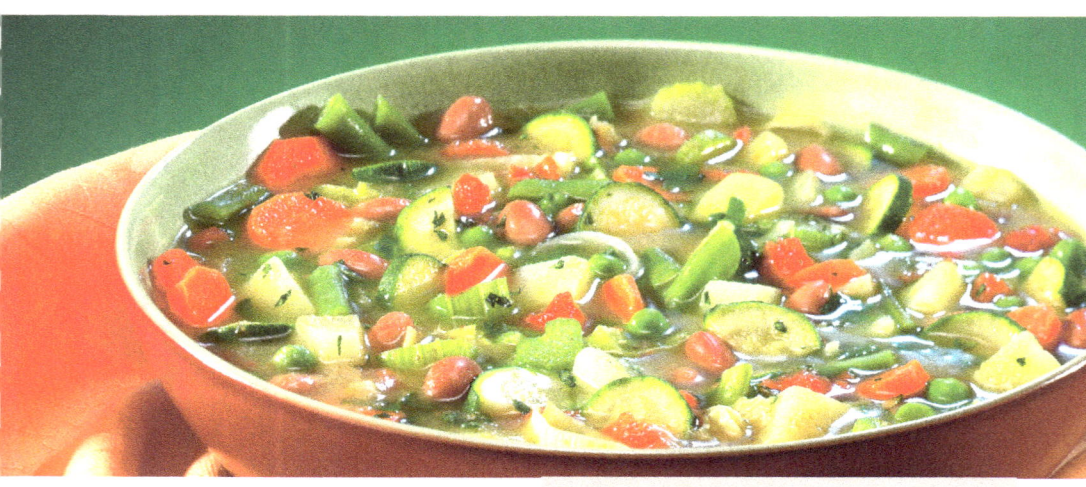

Tinola is a comforting Filipino soup traditionally made with chicken, ginger, and vegetables. This vegetarian version features a variety of fresh vegetables like green papaya or chayote, and spinach, simmered in a flavorful ginger broth. It's a nourishing dish that embodies warmth and home, perfect for family gatherings or a cozy meal.

Author's Personal Connection

Tinola was a staple in our family, especially during the cooler months. My mother would often prepare it when someone was feeling under the weather, believing in its healing properties. The aroma of ginger and fresh vegetables wafting through the house always brought a sense of comfort and home. Now, I enjoy making this vegetarian version for my daughters, sharing the warmth and love that this dish represents in our family.

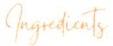
Ingredients

For the Broth
- 1 tablespoon vegetable oil
- 1 medium onion, sliced
- 4 cloves garlic, minced
- 1 tablespoon fresh ginger, sliced
- 1 medium tomato, quartered
- 1 medium green papaya or chayote, peeled and sliced
- 1 cup mushrooms (shiitake or button), sliced
- 4 cups vegetable broth or water
- 2 tablespoons soy sauce
- 1 teaspoon salt (or to taste)
- 1/2 teaspoon black pepper
- 2-3 cups fresh spinach or water spinach (kangkong)
- 1-2 green chili peppers (optional, for a bit of heat)

Servings:	4-6
Preparation Time:	15 min.
Cooking Time:	30 min.
Total Time:	45 min.

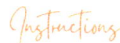
Nutrition:

Calories	150
Protein	5 g
Fat	3 g
Carbohydrates	25 g
Fiber	4 g
Sodium	600 mg

Instructions

Sauté the Aromatics
- In a large pot, heat the vegetable oil over medium heat. Add the sliced onions, minced garlic, and sliced ginger, sautéing until fragrant and the onions become translucent.

Add the Tomatoes
- Stir in the quartered tomatoes and cook until they soften, about 3-4 minutes.

Prepare the Broth
- Add the sliced green papaya or chayote and mushrooms to the pot. Pour in the vegetable broth or water and bring to a boil. Reduce the heat and let it simmer for about 10-15 minutes until the vegetables start to soften.

Season the Soup
- Add the soy sauce, salt, and black pepper. If using, stir in the green chili peppers for a bit of heat.

Finish with Greens
- Add the spinach or water spinach and cook for an additional 2-3 minutes until the greens are wilted.

Serve
- Taste and adjust the seasoning as needed. Serve hot with steamed rice.

Vegetarian Kare-Kare

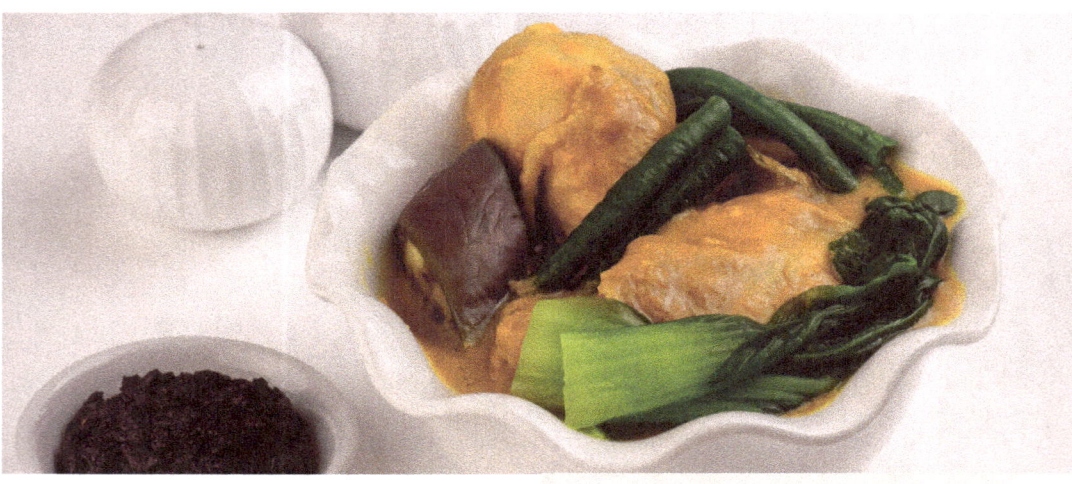

Vegetarian Kare-Kare is a hearty and flavorful peanut stew that showcases a colorful array of vegetables like eggplant, string beans, and banana heart (puso ng saging). This vegetarian adaptation maintains the rich, creamy peanut sauce that Kare-Kare is known for, making it a comforting and satisfying dish perfect for any occasion.

Author's Personal Connection

Kare-Kare has always been a centerpiece during family celebrations in our home. I remember my mother's meticulous preparation of this dish, spending hours to ensure the peanut sauce was just right. The aroma of simmering vegetables and peanut butter would fill the house, drawing everyone to the table. Now, I cherish the opportunity to create this vegetarian version for my daughters, sharing with them the rich flavors and memories tied to this iconic dish.

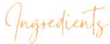

Ingredients

For the Stew

- 2 tablespoons vegetable oil
- 1 medium onion, chopped
- 4 cloves garlic, minced
- 1 medium tomato, chopped
- 1 cup eggplant, sliced into rounds
- 1 cup string beans (sitaw), cut into 2-inch lengths
- 1 cup banana heart (puso ng saging), sliced (optional)
- 1 cup bok choy or water spinach (kangkong)
- 1/2 cup roasted peanuts, ground (or peanut butter)
- 2 cups vegetable broth
- 2 tablespoons soy sauce
- 1 teaspoon salt (to taste)
- 1/2 teaspoon black pepper
- 1 tablespoon annatto powder (for color, optional)

Servings:	4-6
Preparation Time:	20 min.
Cooking Time:	30 min.
Total Time:	50 min.

Nutrition:	
Calories	280
Protein	10 g
Fat	14 g
Carbohydrates	30 g
Fiber	5 g
Sodium	600 mg

Instructions

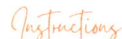

Sauté the Aromatics
- In a large pot, heat the vegetable oil over medium heat. Add the chopped onion and minced garlic, sautéing until fragrant and the onions are translucent.

Add the Tomatoes
- Stir in the chopped tomatoes and cook until they soften, about 3-4 minutes.

Add the Vegetables
- Add the sliced eggplant, string beans, and banana heart (if using) to the pot. Stir well to combine and cook for about 5 minutes.

Prepare the Peanut Sauce
- In a bowl, mix the ground peanuts (or peanut butter) with vegetable broth until smooth. Pour this mixture into the pot along with the soy sauce, salt, black pepper, and annatto powder (if using). Stir to incorporate all the ingredients.

Simmer the Stew
- Bring the mixture to a gentle simmer, cover the pot, and cook for about 15 minutes, or until the vegetables are tender. If the stew is too thick, add more vegetable broth to reach your desired consistency.

Finish with Greens
- Stir in the bok choy or water spinach and cook for an additional 2-3 minutes until the greens are wilted.

Serve
- Taste and adjust the seasoning as needed. Serve hot with steamed rice and a side of bagoong (fermented shrimp paste) or a vegetarian alternative if desired.

Mechado

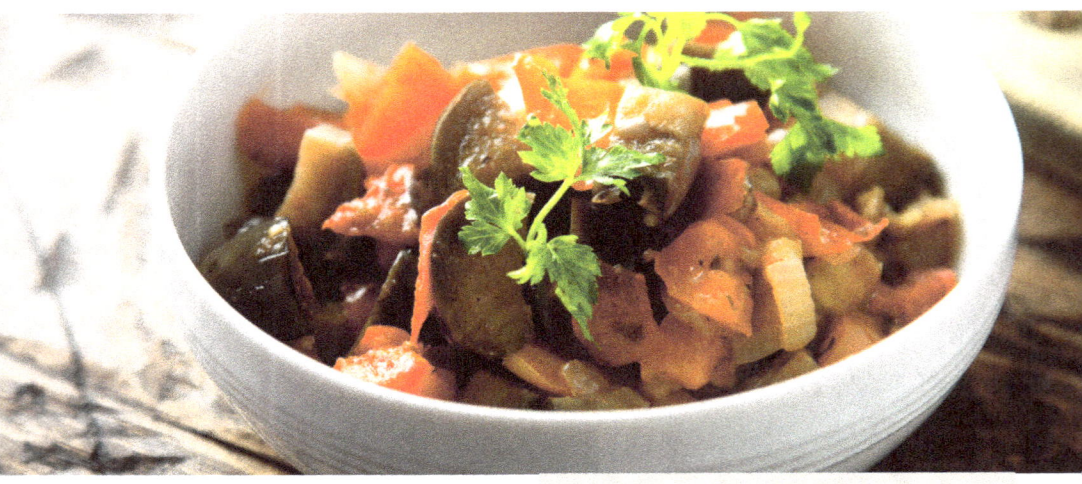

Vegetarian Mechado is a flavorful stew that features a medley of hearty vegetables like potatoes, carrots, and bell peppers, simmered in a rich tomato sauce. This plant-based adaptation retains the deep flavors of the original dish, making it a perfect comfort food that can be enjoyed by everyone.

Mechado was a staple dish in our family, often prepared during special occasions and gatherings. I remember the way my mother would slowly simmer the beef until it was melt-in-your-mouth tender, and the aroma of tomatoes and spices would fill our home. Now, I love to recreate this comforting dish with a vegetarian twist, sharing the same warmth and flavors with my daughters while introducing them to our culinary heritage.

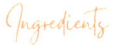
Ingredients

For the Stew
- 2 tablespoons vegetable oil
- 1 medium onion, chopped
- 4 cloves garlic, minced
- 1 medium tomato, chopped
- 2 medium potatoes, peeled and cubed
- 2 medium carrots, sliced
- 1 bell pepper (red or green), sliced
- 1 cup green peas (fresh or frozen)
- 1 cup mushrooms (shiitake or button), sliced
- 2 cups vegetable broth
- 1 can (14 oz) diced tomatoes (or 2 cups fresh tomatoes, chopped)
- 2 tablespoons soy sauce
- 1 tablespoon tomato paste
- 1 teaspoon paprika
- 1/2 teaspoon black pepper
- 1 teaspoon salt (to taste)
- 1 bay leaf
- Fresh parsley or cilantro for garnish (optional)

Servings:	4-6
Preparation Time:	15 min.
Cooking Time:	40 min.
Total Time:	55 min.

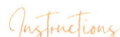
Nutrition:

Calories	220
Protein	6 g
Fat	7 g
Carbohydrates	35 g
Fiber	7 g
Sodium	500 mg

Instructions

Sauté the Aromatics
- In a large pot, heat the vegetable oil over medium heat. Add the chopped onion and minced garlic, sautéing until fragrant and the onions become translucent.

Add the Tomatoes
- Stir in the chopped tomatoes and cook until they soften, about 3-4 minutes.

Add the Vegetables
- Add the cubed potatoes, sliced carrots, and bell pepper to the pot. Stir well to combine and cook for about 5 minutes.

Prepare the Sauce
- Add the vegetable broth, diced tomatoes, soy sauce, tomato paste, paprika, black pepper, salt, and bay leaf. Stir to incorporate all the ingredients.

Simmer the Stew
- Bring the mixture to a boil, then reduce the heat to low. Cover the pot and let it simmer for about 25-30 minutes, or until the vegetables are tender. Stir occasionally, and add water or more broth if the stew becomes too thick.

Finish with Greens
- In the last 5 minutes of cooking, stir in the green peas and sliced mushrooms. Cook until heated through and the mushrooms are tender.

Serve
- Taste and adjust the seasoning as needed. Remove the bay leaf before serving. Garnish with fresh parsley or cilantro if desired. Serve hot with steamed rice.

Filipino Vegetable Curry

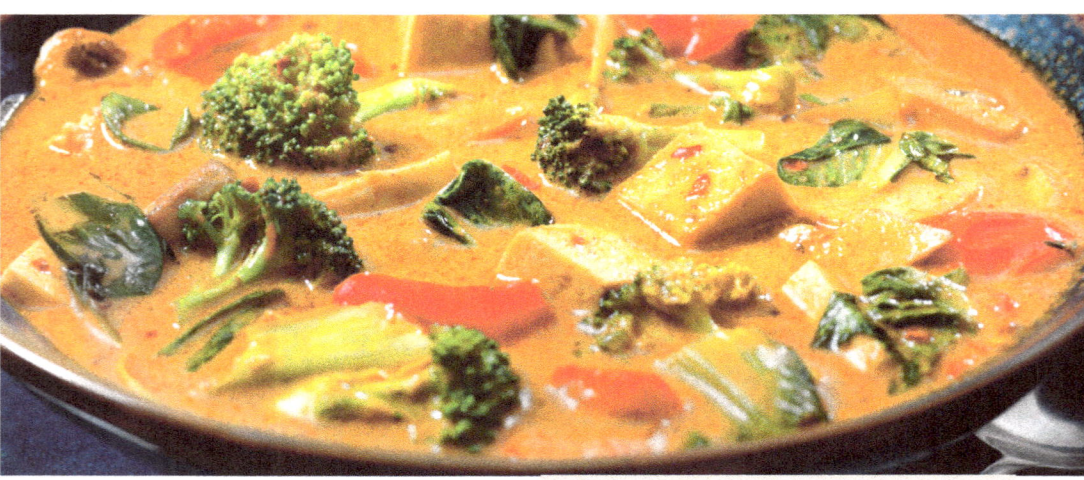

Filipino Vegetable Curry is a vibrant and aromatic dish that features a medley of fresh vegetables simmered in a creamy coconut milk and curry sauce. This comforting dish showcases the unique blend of spices and flavors that Filipino cuisine is known for, making it a perfect meal for any occasion.

Author's Personal Connection

Growing up, our family enjoyed a variety of curries, often featuring whatever vegetables were in season. I remember the warmth and comfort of a steaming bowl of curry, especially on rainy days. The aroma of spices and coconut milk wafting through the kitchen always made me feel at home. Now, I love cooking this Filipino Vegetable Curry for my daughters, sharing the heartwarming flavors of my childhood and encouraging them to appreciate the bounty of fresh produce.

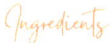
Ingredients

For the Curry

- 2 tablespoons vegetable oil
- 1 medium onion, chopped
- 4 cloves garlic, minced
- 1 tablespoon fresh ginger, minced
- 1-2 tablespoons curry powder (adjust to taste)
- 1 medium carrot, sliced
- 1 cup eggplant, diced
- 1 cup bell peppers (red and green), sliced
- 1 cup green beans (sitaw), trimmed and cut into 2-inch pieces
- 1 can (14 oz) coconut milk
- 1 cup vegetable broth or water
- 2 tablespoons soy sauce
- Salt and black pepper to taste
- 1-2 tablespoons fish sauce (optional, for depth of flavor, or use a vegan alternative)
- Fresh basil or cilantro for garnish (optional)

Servings:	4-6
Preparation Time:	15 min.
Cooking Time:	30 min.
Total Time:	45 min.

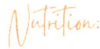
Nutrition:

Calories	250
Protein	5 g
Fat	15 g
Carbohydrates	30 g
Fiber	5 g
Sodium	600 mg

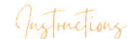
Instructions

Sauté the Aromatics

- In a large pot or deep skillet, heat the vegetable oil over medium heat. Add the chopped onion, minced garlic, and minced ginger, sautéing until fragrant and the onions are translucent.

Add the Spices

- Stir in the curry powder and cook for about 1 minute to toast the spices.

Add the Vegetables

- Add the sliced carrots, diced eggplant, bell peppers, and green beans to the pot. Stir well to coat the vegetables with the spices and sauté for about 5 minutes.

Add the Liquid

- Pour in the coconut milk and vegetable broth (or water). Stir to combine, then bring the mixture to a gentle simmer.

Season the Curry

- Add the soy sauce and fish sauce (if using). Season with salt and black pepper to taste. Let the curry simmer for about 15-20 minutes, or until the vegetables are tender and the flavors meld together.

Serve

- Taste and adjust the seasoning as needed. Serve hot over steamed rice and garnish with fresh basil or cilantro if desired.

Humba

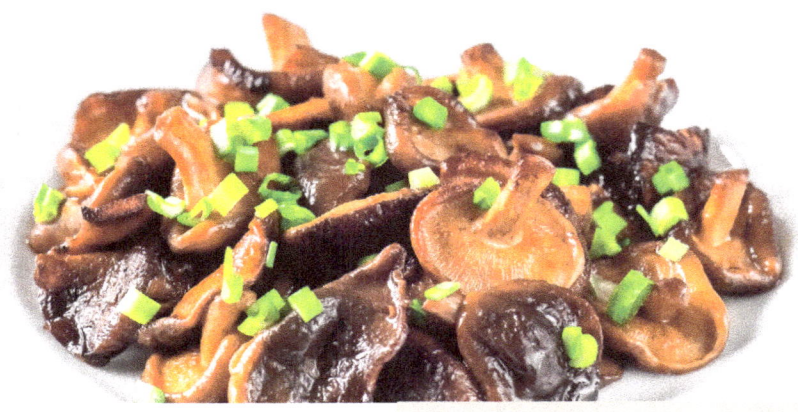

Vegetarian Humba is a savory and rich stew that features a medley of vegetables simmered in a flavorful sauce made from soy sauce, vinegar, and spices. This plant-based adaptation maintains the deep, comforting flavors of the original dish, making it perfect for serving over rice.

Author's Personal Connection

Humba has always been a cherished dish in our family, often prepared during special gatherings and celebrations. I remember the enticing aroma that filled our home as my mother slow-cooked the pork until it was tender and flavorful. Now, I enjoy making this vegetarian version for my daughters, sharing the warmth and love that this dish represents while introducing them to the vibrant flavors of our culinary heritage.

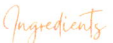

For the Stew

- 2 tablespoons vegetable oil
- 1 medium onion, sliced
- 4 cloves garlic, minced
- 1 medium tomato, chopped
- 1 cup mushrooms (shiitake or button), sliced
- 1 cup eggplant, diced
- 1 cup green beans (sitaw), trimmed
- 1 cup potatoes, peeled and cubed
- 2 tablespoons soy sauce
- 2 tablespoons vinegar (white or cane vinegar)
- 1 tablespoon brown sugar (or coconut sugar)
- 1/2 teaspoon black pepper
- 1 bay leaf
- 1 cup vegetable broth or water
- Salt to taste
- Chopped green onions for garnish (optional)

Servings:	4-6
Preparation Time:	15 min.
Cooking Time:	40 min.
Total Time:	55 min.

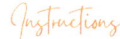

Calories	220
Protein	6 g
Fat	5 g
Carbohydrates	38 g
Fiber	7 g
Sodium	600 mg

Instructions

Sauté the Aromatics

- In a large pot, heat the vegetable oil over medium heat. Add the sliced onions and minced garlic, sautéing until fragrant and the onions become translucent.

Add the Tomatoes

- Stir in the chopped tomatoes and cook until they soften, about 3-4 minutes.

Add the Vegetables

- Add the sliced mushrooms, diced eggplant, green beans, and cubed potatoes to the pot. Stir well to combine and cook for about 5 minutes.

Prepare the Sauce

- Add the soy sauce, vinegar, brown sugar, black pepper, bay leaf, and vegetable broth (or water). Stir to incorporate all the ingredients.

Simmer the Stew

- Bring the mixture to a gentle boil, then reduce the heat to low. Cover the pot and let it simmer for about 25-30 minutes, or until the vegetables are tender. Stir occasionally and add more water if needed.

Finish and Serve

- Taste and adjust the seasoning with salt if needed. Remove the bay leaf before serving. Garnish with chopped green onions if desired. Serve hot with steamed rice.

Vegetarian Bicol Express

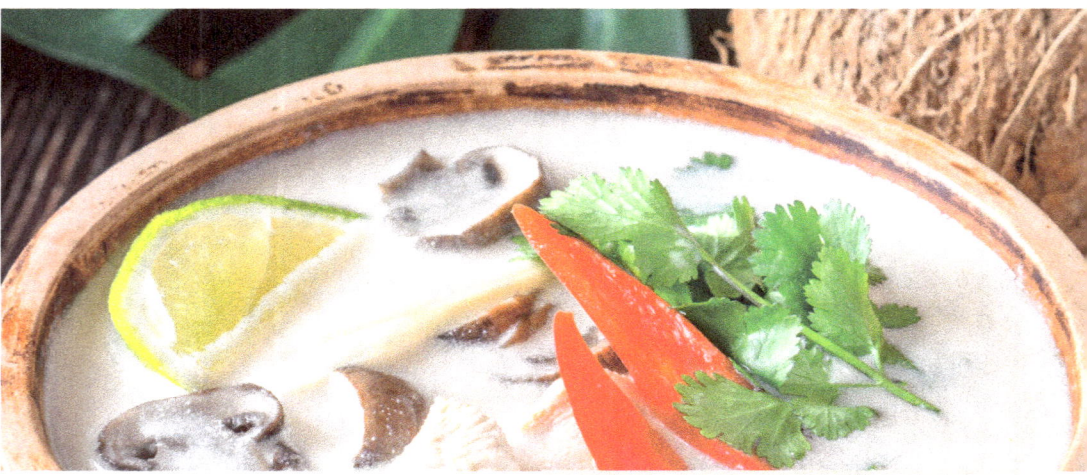

Vegetarian Bicol Express is a creamy and spicy stew made with a variety of vegetables, simmered in rich coconut milk and seasoned with chili peppers. This plant-based adaptation maintains the bold flavors of the original dish while providing a hearty and satisfying meal perfect for rice lovers.

Author's Personal Connection

Bicol Express has always been a favorite in our family, especially for its unique combination of spice and creaminess. I remember my mother preparing this dish during family gatherings, with the aroma of coconut milk and spices wafting through the house. Now, as I make this vegetarian version for my daughters, I hope to pass on the love and warmth that this dish represents, while also introducing them to the vibrant flavors of our culinary heritage.

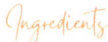

For the Stew

- 2 tablespoons vegetable oil
- 1 medium onion, chopped
- 4 cloves garlic, minced
- 1 tablespoon fresh ginger, minced
- 2-3 Thai chili peppers (or to taste), sliced
- 1 cup eggplant, diced
- 1 cup green beans (sitaw), trimmed and cut into 2-inch pieces
- 1 cup bell peppers (red and green), sliced
- 1 cup mushrooms (shiitake or button), sliced
- 1 can (14 oz) coconut milk
- 2 tablespoons soy sauce
- 1 tablespoon miso paste (for umami flavor)
- Salt and black pepper to taste
- 1-2 tablespoons chili paste or sriracha (optional, for extra heat)
- Fresh basil or cilantro for garnish (optional)

Servings:	4-6
Preparation Time:	15 min.
Cooking Time:	30 min.
Total Time:	45 min.

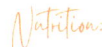

Calories	280
Protein	6 g
Fat	20 g
Carbohydrates	25 g
Fiber	5 g
Sodium	600 mg

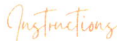

Sauté the Aromatics
- In a large pot or deep skillet, heat the vegetable oil over medium heat. Add the chopped onion, minced garlic, and minced ginger. Sauté until fragrant and the onions become translucent.

Add the Chili Peppers
- Stir in the sliced Thai chili peppers and cook for about 1 minute to release their heat.

Add the Vegetables
- Add the diced eggplant, green beans, bell peppers, and mushrooms to the pot. Stir well to combine and cook for about 5 minutes, allowing the vegetables to soften slightly.

Prepare the Coconut Sauce
- Pour in the coconut milk and add the soy sauce and miso paste. Stir to combine and bring the mixture to a gentle simmer.

Season the Stew
- Season with salt and black pepper to taste. If you prefer a spicier dish, add chili paste or sriracha at this stage. Let the stew simmer for about 15-20 minutes, or until the vegetables are tender and the sauce has thickened.

Serve
- Taste and adjust the seasoning as needed. Serve hot over steamed rice and garnish with fresh basil or cilantro if desired.

Sopas

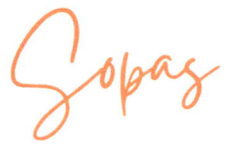

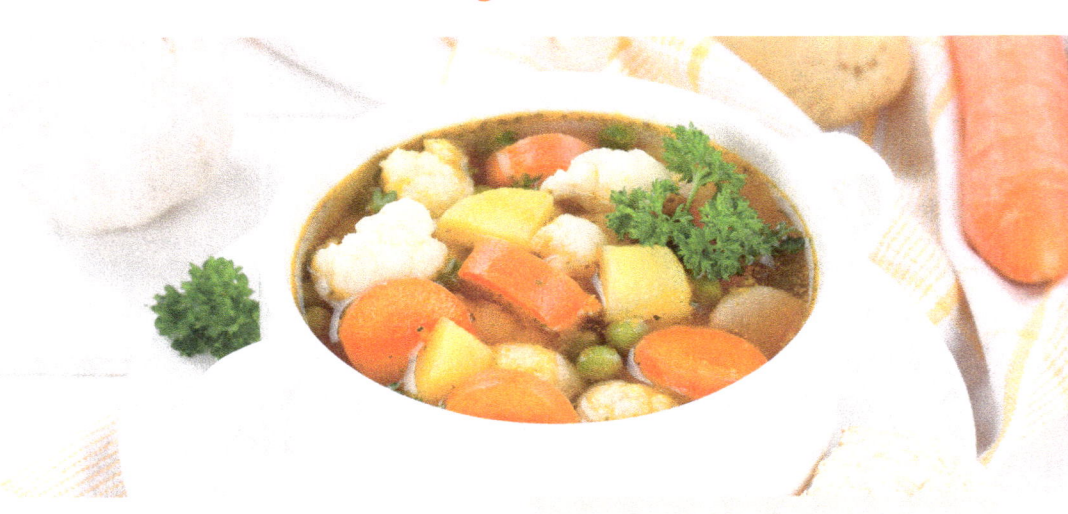

Vegetarian Sopas is a creamy and savory noodle soup that features macaroni, vegetables, and a rich broth. This comforting dish is perfect for any occasion, combining the heartiness of pasta with the warmth of a flavorful soup, making it a beloved meal for families.

Author's Personal Connection

Sopas has always been a staple in our household, especially during the cooler months or when someone was feeling under the weather. I remember my mother's soothing voice as she stirred the pot, filling our home with the comforting aroma of broth and spices. Making this vegetarian version for my daughters allows me to share the same warmth and love that this dish represents, while also providing a healthier, plant-based alternative.

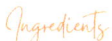

Ingredients

For the Soup

- 2 tablespoons vegetable oil
- 1 medium onion, chopped
- 4 cloves garlic, minced
- 1 medium carrot, diced
- 1 cup celery, diced
- 1 medium potato, peeled and cubed
- 1 cup green beans (sitaw), cut into 1-inch pieces
- 1 cup corn kernels (fresh or frozen)
- 4 cups vegetable broth
- 1 cup water (or more, as needed)
- 1-2 cups elbow macaroni or any pasta of your choice
- 1 cup plant-based milk (coconut milk or almond milk work well)
- Salt and black pepper to taste
- Fresh parsley or green onions for garnish (optional)

Servings:	**4-6**
Preparation Time:	**10 min.**
Cooking Time:	**30 min.**
Total Time:	**40 min.**

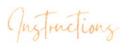

Nutrition:

Calories	**220**
Protein	**6 g**
Fat	**5 g**
Carbohydrates	**38 g**
Fiber	**5 g**
Sodium	**500 mg**

Instructions

Sauté the Aromatics

- In a large pot, heat the vegetable oil over medium heat. Add the chopped onion and minced garlic, sautéing until fragrant and the onions become translucent.

Add the Vegetables

- Stir in the diced carrots, celery, and potatoes. Cook for about 5 minutes, allowing the vegetables to soften slightly.

Add the Broth

- Pour in the vegetable broth and water, bringing the mixture to a boil. Add the green beans and corn, and let it simmer for about 10 minutes.

Cook the Pasta

- Add the elbow macaroni to the pot and cook according to package instructions, usually about 8-10 minutes, until al dente.

Finish with Creaminess

- Once the pasta is cooked, stir in the plant-based milk. Allow the soup to simmer for another 5 minutes, letting the flavors meld together.

Season and Serve

- Taste and adjust the seasoning with salt and black pepper as needed. Serve hot, garnished with fresh parsley or chopped green onions if desired.

Arroz Caldo

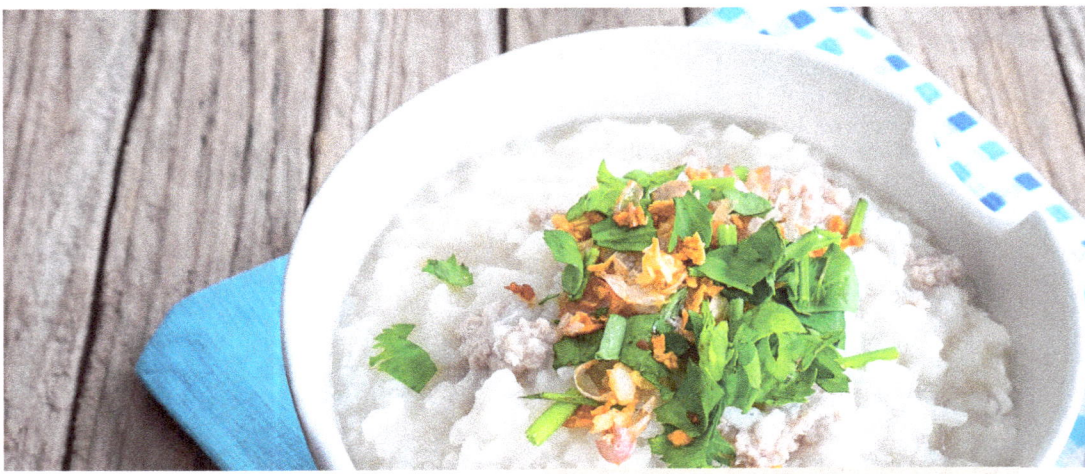

Vegetarian Arroz Caldo is a creamy and soothing rice porridge that features a delightful blend of ginger, garlic, and vegetables. This hearty dish is perfect for cold days or when you're feeling under the weather, offering warmth and comfort with every spoonful.

Author's Personal Connection

Arroz Caldo has always been a cherished comfort food in our family. I remember my mother making it on rainy days or when someone was sick, filling the house with the comforting aroma of ginger and garlic. Preparing this vegetarian version for my daughters allows me to share the same warmth and love that this dish represents, while also introducing them to the flavors of our culture.

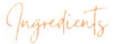
Ingredients

For the Porridge
- 2 tablespoons vegetable oil
- 1 medium onion, chopped
- 4 cloves garlic, minced
- 1 tablespoon fresh ginger, minced
- 1 cup jasmine rice or any rice of your choice
- 6 cups vegetable broth or water
- 1 cup carrots, diced
- 1 cup celery, diced
- 1 cup green beans (sitaw), cut into 1-inch pieces
- 1 cup corn kernels (fresh or frozen)
- 2-3 tablespoons soy sauce (adjust to taste)
- Salt and black pepper to taste
- Chopped green onions and/or fried garlic for garnish
- Lemon or calamansi wedges for serving (optional)

Servings:	4-6
Preparation Time:	10 min.
Cooking Time:	30 min.
Total Time:	40 min.

Nutrition:

Calories	200
Protein	5 g
Fat	4 g
Carbohydrates	38 g
Fiber	5 g
Sodium	600 mg

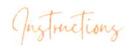
Instructions

Sauté the Aromatics
- In a large pot, heat the vegetable oil over medium heat. Add the chopped onion, minced garlic, and minced ginger, sautéing until fragrant and the onions become translucent.

Add the Rice
- Stir in the jasmine rice and cook for about 1-2 minutes, allowing the rice to soak up the flavors.

Add the Broth
- Pour in the vegetable broth or water, bringing the mixture to a boil. Reduce the heat to low and let it simmer, covered, for about 20 minutes, stirring occasionally, until the rice is cooked and the porridge reaches your desired consistency.

Add the Vegetables
- Stir in the diced carrots, celery, green beans, and corn. Continue to simmer for another 5-10 minutes until the vegetables are tender.

Season the Porridge
- Add the soy sauce, salt, and black pepper to taste. Adjust the seasoning according to your preference.

Serve
- Ladle the Arroz Caldo into bowls and garnish with chopped green onions and fried garlic. Serve hot with lemon or calamansi wedges on the side for an extra kick.

Adobo sa Gata

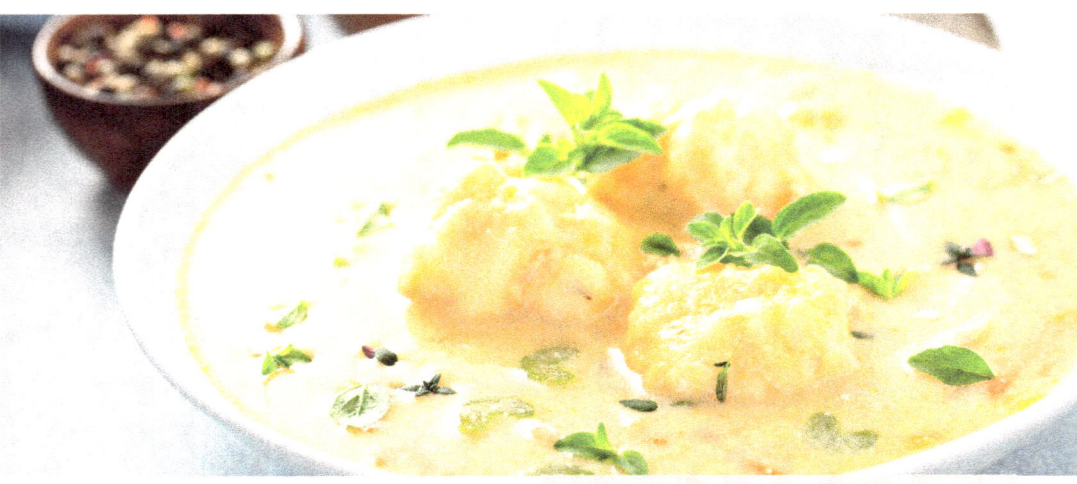

Vegetarian Adobo sa Gata is a rich and aromatic stew that features a medley of vegetables simmered in a savory coconut milk sauce infused with garlic, vinegar, and soy sauce. This comforting dish captures the essence of traditional Filipino adobo while providing a plant-based alternative that's both hearty and satisfying.

Author's Personal Connection

Adobo sa Gata has always been one of my favorite Filipino dishes, celebrated for its unique blend of flavors. I fondly remember my mother preparing it during family gatherings, with the aroma of garlic and coconut filling our home. Making this vegetarian version allows me to share the same warmth and love with my daughters while introducing them to the comforting flavors of our heritage.

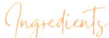

Ingredients

For the Stew
- 2 tablespoons vegetable oil
- 1 medium onion, sliced
- 4 cloves garlic, minced
- 1 tablespoon fresh ginger, minced (optional)
- 1 cup mushrooms (shiitake or button), sliced
- 1 medium eggplant, sliced into rounds
- 1 cup green beans (sitaw), trimmed and cut into 2-inch pieces
- 1 medium potato, peeled and cubed
- 1 can (14 oz) coconut milk
- 1/4 cup soy sauce
- 1/4 cup vinegar (cane or white vinegar)
- 1-2 tablespoons brown sugar (or coconut sugar)
- 1 teaspoon black pepper
- 1 bay leaf
- Salt to taste
- Fresh cilantro or green onions for garnish (optional)

Servings:	**4-6**
Preparation Time:	**15 min.**
Cooking Time:	**30 min.**
Total Time:	**45 min.**

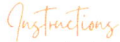

Nutrition:

Calories	**280**
Protein	**6 g**
Fat	**20 g**
Carbohydrates	**25 g**
Fiber	**5 g**
Sodium	**600 mg**

Instructions

Sauté the Aromatics
- In a large pot, heat the vegetable oil over medium heat. Add the sliced onion and minced garlic, sautéing until fragrant and the onions are translucent.

Add the Vegetables
- Stir in the minced ginger (if using), mushrooms, and eggplant. Cook for about 5 minutes, allowing the vegetables to soften slightly.

Add the Remaining Ingredients
- Add the cubed potato, green beans, coconut milk, soy sauce, vinegar, brown sugar, black pepper, and bay leaf. Stir well to combine all the ingredients.

Simmer the Stew
- Bring the mixture to a gentle simmer. Cover the pot and let it cook for about 20-25 minutes, or until the vegetables are tender and the flavors meld together. Stir occasionally, and add a little water if the sauce becomes too thick.

Season and Serve
- Taste and adjust the seasoning with salt if needed. Remove the bay leaf before serving. Garnish with fresh cilantro or chopped green onions if desired. Serve hot with steamed rice.

Bulalo

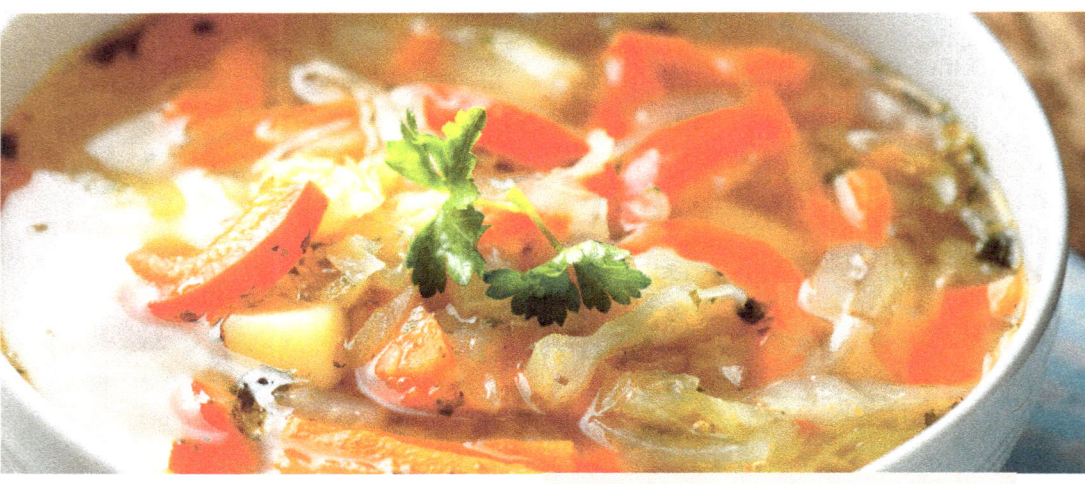

Vegetarian Bulalo is a comforting and hearty vegetable soup that features a rich broth infused with a blend of spices and fresh vegetables. While the original Bulalo is known for its tender beef and marrow, this vegetarian version uses hearty vegetables and plant-based ingredients to create a satisfying and nourishing dish.

Author's Personal Connection

Bulalo has always been a beloved dish in our family, especially enjoyed during family gatherings and celebrations. I remember the warmth of the soup and the joy of sharing it with loved ones around the table. Making this vegetarian version allows me to pass on the flavors of my childhood while providing a healthier, plant-based alternative that my daughters can enjoy.

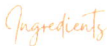
Ingredients

For the Broth
- 2 tablespoons vegetable oil
- 1 medium onion, quartered
- 4 cloves garlic, minced
- 1 tablespoon fresh ginger, sliced
- 1 medium carrot, sliced into rounds
- 1 medium potato, peeled and cubed
- 1 cup corn (fresh or frozen)
- 1 cup green beans (sitaw), trimmed and cut into 2-inch pieces
- 1 cup cabbage, chopped
- 6 cups vegetable broth or water
- 2 tablespoons soy sauce
- 1 tablespoon miso paste (optional, for added umami flavor)
- 1-2 pieces star anise (optional, for flavor)
- Salt and black pepper to taste
- Chopped green onions for garnish (optional)

Servings:	4-6
Preparation Time:	15 min.
Cooking Time:	40 min.
Total Time:	55 min.

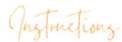
Nutrition:

Calories	180
Protein	5 g
Fat	3 g
Carbohydrates	35 g
Fiber	6 g
Sodium	600 mg

Instructions

Sauté the Aromatics
- In a large pot, heat the vegetable oil over medium heat. Add the quartered onion, minced garlic, and sliced ginger. Sauté until fragrant and the onions become translucent.

Add the Vegetables
- Stir in the sliced carrots and cubed potatoes. Cook for about 5 minutes, allowing the vegetables to soften slightly.

Prepare the Broth
- Add the corn, green beans, and chopped cabbage to the pot. Pour in the vegetable broth or water and bring the mixture to a boil.

Season the Soup
- Add the soy sauce, miso paste (if using), and star anise (if using). Season with salt and black pepper to taste. Reduce the heat and let it simmer for about 25-30 minutes, or until the vegetables are tender.

Serve
- Taste and adjust the seasoning as needed. Remove the star anise before serving. Serve hot in bowls, garnished with chopped green onions if desired. This soup is perfect with steamed rice.

RICE AND GRAINS

Garlic Fried Rice

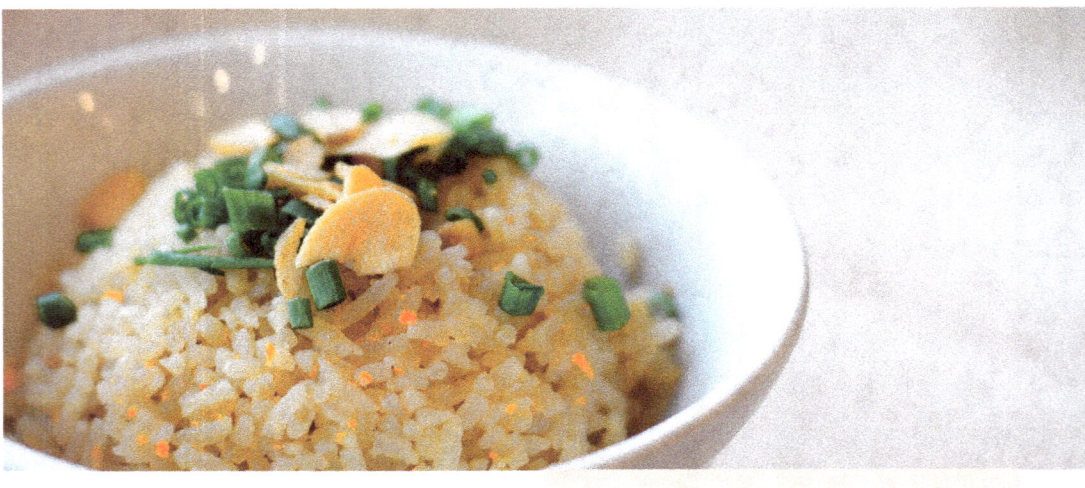

Garlic Fried Rice, or Sinangag, is a flavorful and aromatic dish made from leftover rice sautéed with plenty of garlic. This easy-to-make rice dish is a perfect accompaniment to any meal, adding a delightful crunch and savory flavor that elevates the dining experience.

Author's Personal Connection

Garlic Fried Rice is a breakfast favorite in our household, often enjoyed with eggs or leftover dishes from the night before. I have fond memories of waking up to the enticing aroma of garlic sizzling in the pan, signaling that a delicious meal was on the way. Sharing this simple yet flavorful dish with my daughters allows me to pass down a piece of our culinary heritage, reminding them of the warmth and love found in home-cooked meals.

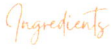
Ingredients

For the Fried Rice
- 4 cups cooked rice (preferably day-old rice for better texture)
- 4 tablespoons vegetable oil
- 6-8 cloves garlic, minced
- 1/2 teaspoon salt (or to taste)
- 1/4 teaspoon black pepper (or to taste)
- 2-3 green onions, chopped (for garnish)
- Optional: 1-2 eggs, scrambled (for added protein, if desired)

Servings:	4
Preparation Time:	5 min.
Cooking Time:	10 min.
Total Time:	15 min.

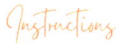
Nutrition:

Calories	220
Protein	4 g
Fat	8 g
Carbohydrates	34 g
Fiber	1 g
Sodium	300 mg

Instructions

Prepare the Rice
- If using refrigerated leftover rice, break up any clumps with your hands or a fork to ensure even frying.

Sauté the Garlic
- In a large skillet or wok, heat the vegetable oil over medium heat. Add the minced garlic and sauté until golden brown and fragrant, being careful not to burn it (about 2-3 minutes).

Add the Rice
- Add the cooked rice to the skillet, stirring well to coat the rice with the garlic and oil. Cook for about 5-7 minutes, stirring frequently, until the rice is heated through and slightly crispy.

Season
- Season the rice with salt and black pepper to taste. If using, push the rice to one side of the skillet and scramble the eggs in the empty space until fully cooked, then mix them into the rice.

Garnish and Serve
- Remove the skillet from heat and garnish the Garlic Fried Rice with chopped green onions. Serve hot as a side dish or as a main meal.

Coconut Rice

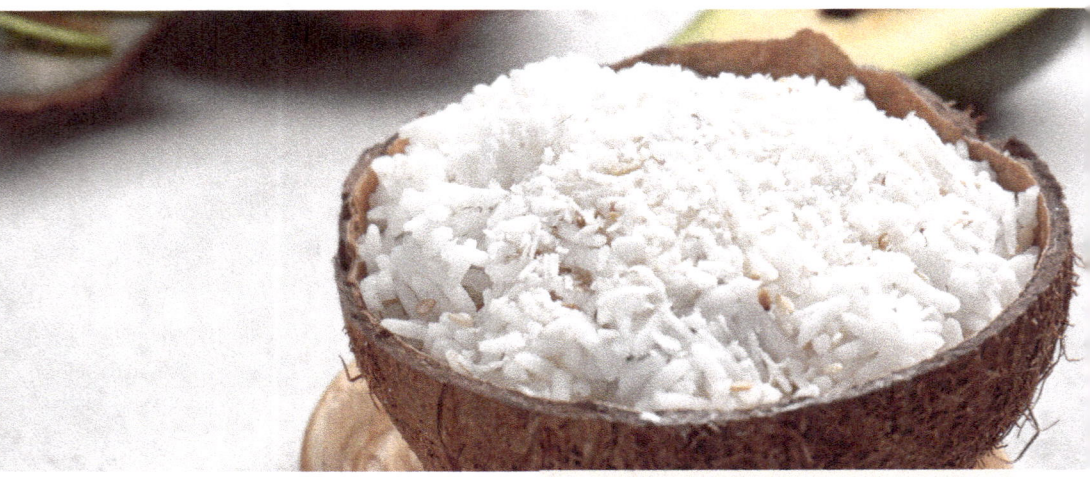

Coconut Rice is a fragrant and creamy rice dish made by cooking rice in coconut milk, which imparts a subtle sweetness and rich flavor. This dish is perfect for accompanying savory meals or can be enjoyed on its own as a comforting side.

Author's Personal Connection

Coconut Rice has always been a special treat in our family, often prepared during celebrations or special occasions. I remember the excitement of watching my mother cook the rice, filling our home with the enticing aroma of coconut. Sharing this dish with my daughters allows me to pass on the flavors of our heritage and create new memories around the dining table.

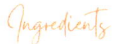
Ingredients

For the Fried Rice
- 4 cups cooked rice (preferably day-old rice for better texture)
- 4 tablespoons vegetable oil
- 6-8 cloves garlic, minced
- 1/2 teaspoon salt (or to taste)
- 1/4 teaspoon black pepper (or to taste)
- 2-3 green onions, chopped (for garnish)
- Optional: 1-2 eggs, scrambled (for added protein, if desired)

Servings:	**4**
Preparation Time:	**5 min.**
Cooking Time:	**25 min.**
Total Time:	**30 min.**

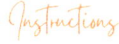
Nutrition:

Calories	**250**
Protein	**4 g**
Fat	**9 g**
Carbohydrates	**40 g**
Fiber	**2 g**
Sodium	**300 mg**

Instructions

Rinse the Rice
- Rinse the jasmine rice under cold water until the water runs clear to remove excess starch. Drain well.

Combine Ingredients
- In a medium saucepan, combine the rinsed rice, coconut milk, water, salt, and sugar (if using). If you have pandan leaves, tie them in a knot and add them to the pot for extra fragrance.

Cook the Rice
- Bring the mixture to a boil over medium heat. Once it starts boiling, reduce the heat to low, cover the pot, and let it simmer for about 15-20 minutes, or until the rice is cooked and the liquid is absorbed. Avoid lifting the lid during cooking to ensure even cooking.

Fluff and Serve
- Once the rice is cooked, remove the pot from heat and let it sit, covered, for 5 minutes. Fluff the rice with a fork, discarding the pandan leaves if used. Serve warm as a side dish with your favorite Filipino dishes.

SOUPS AND STEWS

Vegetarian Mami

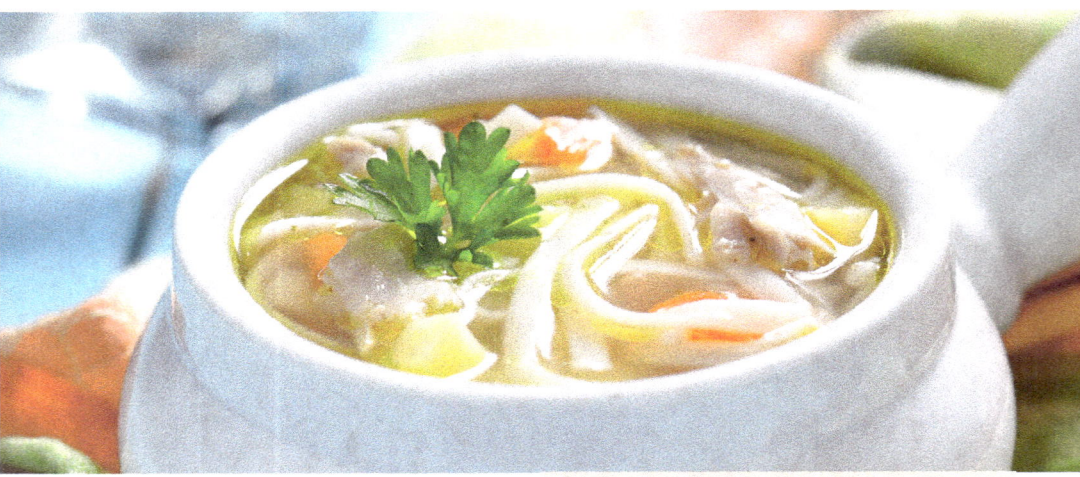

Vegetarian Mami is a warm and hearty noodle soup that features flavorful broth, tender vegetables, and egg noodles. This comforting dish is perfect for chilly days or when you crave a soothing bowl of soup, offering a delicious plant-based alternative to the traditional version.

Author's Personal Connection

Mami has always been a favorite comfort food in our household, especially during rainy days. I remember my mother preparing it with love, filling the house with the enticing aroma of broth and spices. Making this vegetarian version for my daughters allows me to share the warmth and flavors of my childhood while introducing them to the joys of plant-based eating.

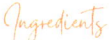

Ingredients

For the Broth
- 2 tablespoons vegetable oil
- 1 medium onion, sliced
- 4 cloves garlic, minced
- 1 tablespoon fresh ginger, minced
- 1 medium carrot, sliced
- 1 cup shiitake mushrooms or button mushrooms, sliced
- 4 cups vegetable broth
- 2 tablespoons soy sauce
- 1 tablespoon miso paste (optional, for added umami flavor)
- Salt and black pepper to taste
- 2-3 green onions, chopped (for garnish)
- 1 cup baby spinach or bok choy (for added greens)

For the Noodles
- 8 oz egg noodles (or any noodles of your choice)
- Optional: boiled eggs (for non-vegetarian version)

Servings:	4
Preparation Time:	10 min.
Cooking Time:	30 min.
Total Time:	40 min.

Nutrition:

Calories	230
Protein	8 g
Fat	5 g
Carbohydrates	40 g
Fiber	4 g
Sodium	600 mg

Instructions

Sauté the Aromatics
- In a large pot, heat the vegetable oil over medium heat. Add the sliced onion, minced garlic, and minced ginger, sautéing until fragrant and the onions become translucent.

Add the Vegetables
- Stir in the sliced carrots and mushrooms. Cook for about 5 minutes until the vegetables are slightly softened.

Prepare the Broth
- Pour in the vegetable broth and bring the mixture to a boil. Add the soy sauce and miso paste (if using). Season with salt and black pepper to taste. Let it simmer for about 15 minutes.

Cook the Noodles
- While the broth is simmering, cook the egg noodles according to package instructions. Drain and set aside.

Finish the Soup
- Add the cooked noodles and baby spinach or bok choy to the broth, stirring until the greens are wilted and everything is heated through.

Serve
- Ladle the Vegetarian Mami into bowls and garnish with chopped green onions. Serve hot, and enjoy!

Vegetarian Sinigang

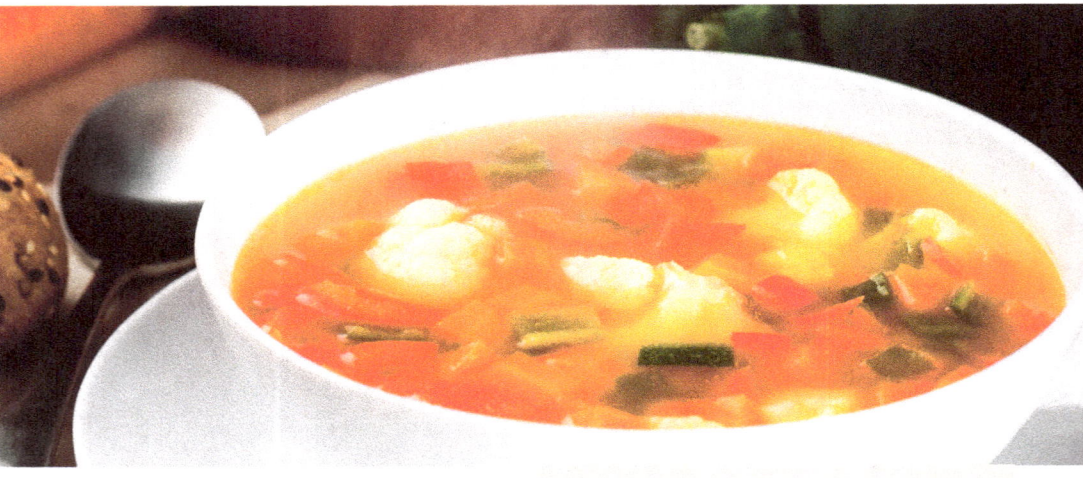

Vegetarian Sinigang is a comforting and tangy soup made with a variety of fresh vegetables simmered in a sour broth. This vegetarian adaptation maintains the signature sour flavor achieved through tamarind or other souring agents while showcasing the natural sweetness of the vegetables, making it a perfect dish for any occasion.

Author's Personal Connection

Sinigang na Baboy was a staple in our family, especially enjoyed during family gatherings and rainy days. The aroma of the sour broth simmering on the stove always brought comfort and warmth to our home. Now, I love making this vegetarian version for my daughters, sharing the same comforting flavors and cherished memories from my childhood.

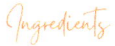 **Ingredients**

For the Broth
- 1 tablespoon vegetable oil
- 1 medium onion, quartered
- 4 cloves garlic, minced
- 1 medium tomato, quartered
- 1 radish (labanos), sliced
- 1 cup eggplant, sliced
- 1 cup green beans (sitaw), cut into 2-inch pieces
- 1 cup water spinach (kangkong) or spinach
- 1 cup water
- 1/2 cup tamarind paste or 1-2 cups fresh tamarind (or use a souring agent like calamansi or green mango)
- 2 tablespoons soy sauce
- 1 teaspoon salt (or to taste)
- 1/2 teaspoon black pepper
- 1-2 green chili peppers (optional, for heat)

Servings:	4-6
Preparation Time:	15 min.
Cooking Time:	30 min.
Total Time:	45 min.

 Nutrition:

Calories	120
Protein	4 g
Fat	3 g
Carbohydrates	20 g
Fiber	5 g
Sodium	600 mg

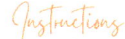 **Instructions**

Sauté the Aromatics
- In a large pot, heat the vegetable oil over medium heat. Add the quartered onions and minced garlic, sautéing until fragrant and the onions become translucent.

Add the Tomatoes
- Stir in the quartered tomatoes and cook until they soften, about 3-4 minutes.

Prepare the Broth
- Add the sliced radish, eggplant, and green beans to the pot. Pour in the water and bring to a boil. Reduce the heat and let it simmer for about 10 minutes until the vegetables begin to soften.

Add the Tamarind
- If using fresh tamarind, boil it in a separate pot with a little water until soft, then mash and strain the juice into the soup. If using tamarind paste, simply add it to the pot and stir well. Adjust the sourness to your preference by adding more tamarind or souring agent.

Season and Finish
- Add the soy sauce, salt, black pepper, and green chili peppers (if using). Stir in the water spinach or spinach and cook for an additional 2-3 minutes until the greens are wilted.

Serve
- Taste and adjust the seasoning as needed. Serve hot over steamed rice.

DESSERTS

Leche Flan

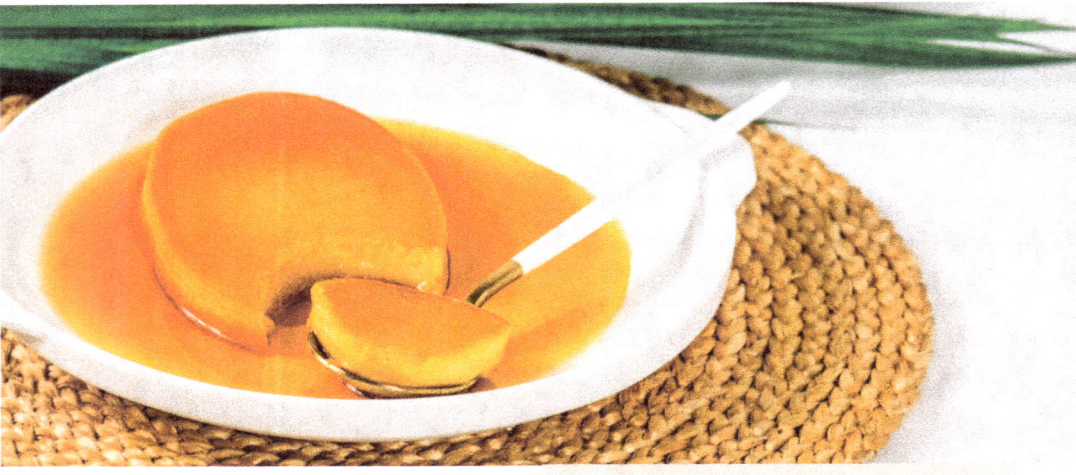

Vegetarian Leche Flan is a decadent Filipino dessert that features a silky smooth custard made with coconut milk and sweetened condensed milk. Topped with a rich caramel sauce, this dessert is perfect for celebrations and family gatherings, offering a delightful twist on the classic flan.

Author's Personal Connection

Leche Flan has always been a highlight at family celebrations and gatherings. I remember my mother carefully preparing this dessert, watching as she poured the rich caramel sauce over the flan. The anticipation of tasting that creamy, sweet goodness was always a treat. Now, I love making this vegetarian version for my daughters, sharing the same joy and sweetness that this dessert brings to our family.

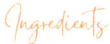
Ingredients

For the Caramel
- 1 cup sugar
- 1/4 cup water

For the Flan
- 1 can (13.5 oz) coconut milk
- 1 can (14 oz) sweetened condensed coconut milk (or regular sweetened condensed milk)
- 4 large eggs
- 1 teaspoon vanilla extract
Pinch of salt

Servings:	**8**
Preparation Time:	**15 min.**
Cooking Time:	**1 hr.**
Total Time:	**1 hr. 15 min.**

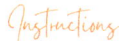
Nutrition:

Calories	**220**
Protein	**4 g**
Fat	**10 g**
Carbohydrates	**30 g**
Fiber	**0 g**
Sodium	**90 mg**

Instructions

Prepare the Caramel
- In a small saucepan, combine the sugar and water over medium heat. Stir until the sugar dissolves, then stop stirring and allow the mixture to boil.
- Cook until the caramel turns a golden amber color. Be careful not to burn it.
- Immediately pour the caramel into a round baking dish or individual ramekins, tilting to coat the bottom evenly. Set aside to cool.

Prepare the Flan
- In a mixing bowl, whisk together the coconut milk, sweetened condensed coconut milk, eggs, vanilla extract, and a pinch of salt until smooth and well combined.
- Strain the mixture through a fine sieve into the prepared caramel-coated dish to ensure a silky texture.

Bake the Flan
- Preheat your oven to 350°F (175°C).
- Place the flan dish in a larger baking pan and fill the outer pan with hot water until it reaches halfway up the sides of the flan dish (this is called a water bath).
- Bake for about 50-60 minutes, or until a knife inserted in the center comes out clean.

Cool and Serve
- Once done, remove the flan from the oven and let it cool at room temperature. Then refrigerate for at least 4 hours or overnight to set.
- To serve, run a knife along the edges of the flan to loosen it. Invert the flan onto a serving plate, allowing the caramel to drizzle over the top.

Bibingka

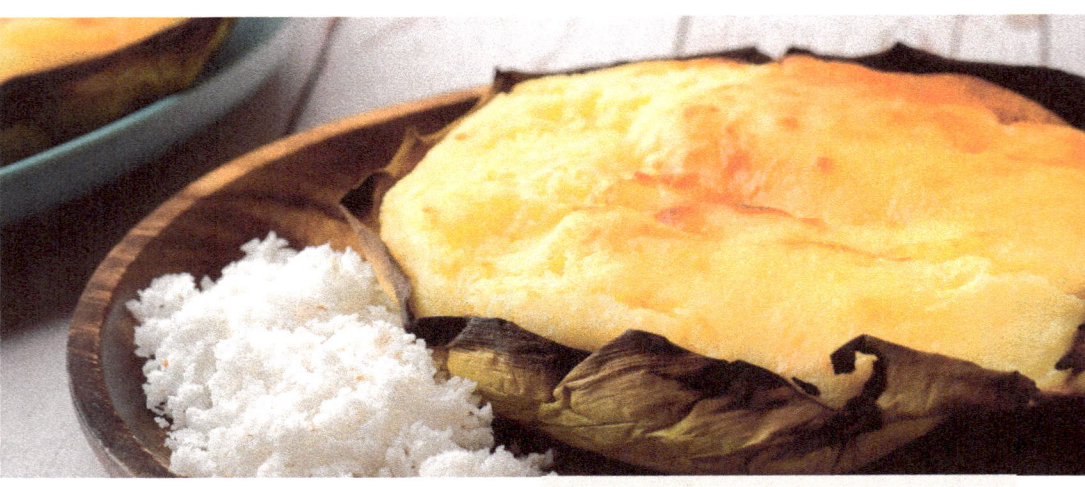

Bibingka is a soft, fluffy rice cake made with rice flour and coconut milk, often baked in banana leaves for added flavor. This delightful treat is traditionally served warm and is usually topped with cheese and salted eggs, making it a favorite during festive occasions.

Author's Personal Connection

Bibingka has always been a cherished part of our family's holiday celebrations. I remember the excitement of attending the early morning Misa de Gallo (Simbang Gabi) and enjoying fresh bibingka sold by street vendors. The warm, sweet aroma of coconut and the soft texture of the cake always filled me with nostalgia. Making this vegetarian version allows me to share these memories with my daughters and create new traditions around this beloved dish.

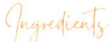
Ingredients

For the Caramel
- 1 cup sugar
- 1/4 cup water

For the Flan
- 1 can (13.5 oz) coconut milk
- 1 can (14 oz) sweetened condensed coconut milk (or regular sweetened condensed milk)
- 4 large eggs
- 1 teaspoon vanilla extract

Pinch of salt

Servings:	**8**
Preparation Time:	**15 min.**
Cooking Time:	**30 min.**
Total Time:	**45 min.**

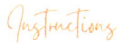
Nutrition:

Calories	**220**
Protein	**4 g**
Fat	**10 g**
Carbohydrates	**30 g**
Fiber	**0 g**
Sodium	**90 mg**

Instructions

Prepare the Caramel
- In a small saucepan, combine the sugar and water over medium heat. Stir until the sugar dissolves, then stop stirring and allow the mixture to boil.
- Cook until the caramel turns a golden amber color. Be careful not to burn it.
- Immediately pour the caramel into a round baking dish or individual ramekins, tilting to coat the bottom evenly. Set aside to cool.

Prepare the Flan
- In a mixing bowl, whisk together the coconut milk, sweetened condensed coconut milk, eggs, vanilla extract, and a pinch of salt until smooth and well combined.
- Strain the mixture through a fine sieve into the prepared caramel-coated dish to ensure a silky texture.

Bake the Flan
- Preheat your oven to 350°F (175°C).
- Place the flan dish in a larger baking pan and fill the outer pan with hot water until it reaches halfway up the sides of the flan dish (this is called a water bath).
- Bake for about 50-60 minutes, or until a knife inserted in the center comes out clean.

Cool and Serve
- Once done, remove the flan from the oven and let it cool at room temperature. Then refrigerate for at least 4 hours or overnight to set.
- To serve, run a knife along the edges of the flan to loosen it. Invert the flan onto a serving plate, allowing the caramel to drizzle over the top.

FILIPINO INGREDIENT SHOPPING MADE SIMPLE

Essential INGREDIENTS FOR FILIPINO VEGETARIAN COOKING

When it comes to Filipino cooking, having the right ingredients on hand can make all the difference in creating authentic and satisfying vegetarian dishes. Here's a handy list of essential ingredients that will elevate your cooking and help you recreate the vibrant flavors of our beloved cuisine:

1. **Rice:** As the staple of Filipino meals, rice is a must-have. Jasmine rice is commonly used, but you can also explore other varieties like brown rice or even sticky rice for special desserts.

2. **Coconut Milk:** This creamy delight is essential for many Filipino dishes, adding richness and depth. Look for canned coconut milk or fresh coconut milk if you're feeling adventurous!

3. **Soy Sauce:** A versatile and savory condiment, soy sauce is used in marinades, stir-fries, and soups. It's an essential ingredient for achieving that umami flavor in your dishes.

4. **Tamarind:** This tangy fruit is key for sour dishes like **Sinigang**. You can find tamarind paste in Asian markets or use fresh tamarind pods if available.

5. **Miso Paste:** This fermented soybean product is fantastic for adding umami to soups and sauces. It's a great substitute for fish sauce in vegetarian recipes.

6. **Fresh Vegetables:** Stock up on a variety of vegetables like eggplant, green beans, bitter melon, radish, and leafy greens such as **kangkong** (water spinach) or **pechay** (bok choy). These will be the stars of your vegetarian dishes!

7. **Spices and Seasonings:** Don't forget spices! Commonly used spices include black pepper, paprika, and chili peppers for that extra kick. Fresh herbs like cilantro and green onions add brightness to your meals.

8. **Plant-Based Proteins:** Tofu, tempeh, and legumes like lentils and chickpeas are great sources of protein and can be used in a variety of dishes. They soak up flavors beautifully and make your meals hearty and satisfying.

WHERE TO FIND FILIPINO VEGETARIAN INGREDIENTS

Now that you know what to look for, the next step is finding these ingredients. Here are some tips on where to shop for Filipino vegetarian essentials:

1. **Asian Grocery Stores:** Your best bet for authentic Filipino ingredients is your local Asian grocery store. These stores often carry a wide range of Filipino products, including rice, sauces, and snacks. Don't be shy to ask the staff for help—they're usually very knowledgeable and can guide you to the right products!
2. **International Markets:** Larger international grocery stores often have a section dedicated to Asian products. You can find staples like soy sauce, coconut milk, and various types of rice here.
3. **Farmers' Markets:** Support your local farmers by visiting farmers' markets for fresh produce. You can often find seasonal vegetables that are perfect for Filipino dishes. Plus, it's a great way to connect with your community!
4. **Online Shopping:** If you're unable to find certain ingredients locally, many Asian grocery items can be purchased online. Websites that specialize in Asian foods often have a wide selection of products available for delivery.
5. **Filipino Restaurants:** Don't forget about local Filipino restaurants! While they may not sell ingredients directly, many chefs are happy to share tips on where to find specific items or even recommend local suppliers.
6. **Community Resources:** Join local Filipino community groups on social media or forums. Members often share tips on where to find specific ingredients, as well as their favorite local markets.

With this guide in hand, you'll be well-equipped to embark on your Filipino vegetarian cooking journey. Embrace the adventure of shopping for ingredients, and remember that each item you gather is a step toward creating delicious meals infused with love and tradition.

CULTURAL CONTEXT AND PERSONAL STORIES

THE ROLE OF FOOD IN FILIPINO CULTURE AND HERITAGE

Food is at the very heart of Filipino culture. It's more than just sustenance; it's a means of connection, a celebration of heritage, and a way to express love. In the Philippines, sharing a meal is an integral part of our social fabric, bringing families and friends together to bond over the flavors and stories that shape our identity.

- **Celebrations and Gatherings:** Filipino culture is rich with festivities, and food plays a central role in these celebrations. Whether it's a birthday, a fiesta, or a holiday, special dishes like **Lechon** (roast pig) or **Pancit** (noodles) take center stage, symbolizing abundance and prosperity. Each dish tells a story and carries memories that connect generations.

- **Family Traditions:** In Filipino households, cooking is often a communal activity. Family members gather in the kitchen, sharing laughter and stories while preparing meals together. These moments create lasting bonds and instill a sense of belonging, where recipes are passed down from one generation to the next.

- **Cultural Identity:** Food is a celebration of our history and diversity. With influences from Malay, Chinese, Spanish, and American cuisines, Filipino food reflects our rich cultural tapestry. Each dish is a testament to our resilience and creativity, showcasing what it means to be Filipino.

In embracing vegetarianism, we have the opportunity to preserve and adapt these cherished culinary traditions. By reimagining beloved recipes, we can continue to celebrate our heritage while making conscious choices that honor our health and the environment.

PERSONAL ANECDOTES FROM JANINE'S KITCHEN

As I reflect on my culinary journey, I'm filled with cherished memories that revolve around food and family. Here are a few anecdotes from my kitchen that highlight the profound connection between cooking and love:

- *Saturday Mornings with Mom:* Growing up, Saturday mornings were reserved for cooking sessions with my mother. We would wake up early, and the aroma of garlic sizzling in oil would greet us as we prepared our favorite breakfast: **Tocino** (sweet cured pork) with garlic fried rice. While we cooked, she would share stories about her childhood in the Philippines, teaching me not just how to cook but also the importance of our culinary heritage.

- *Family Gatherings:* During family reunions, my aunts and uncles would bring their signature dishes, each one a labor of love. I fondly remember my aunt's **Pancit Malabon** and my grandmother's **Sinigang**. We would sit around the table for hours, laughing and sharing stories, the food becoming a backdrop for our connections. These gatherings reinforced the idea that food has the power to bring people together, creating memories that last a lifetime.

- *Cooking for My Daughters:* As a mother, I strive to pass down these traditions to my daughters, Katie and Lovella. I involve them in the kitchen, teaching them the recipes and stories behind each dish. One of their favorites is helping me make **Vegetarian Lumpiang Shanghai**. They love to wrap the spring rolls, and I delight in watching them embrace our culture while adding their unique twist to the recipe. It's a beautiful way to bond and create new memories together.

- *Adapting Recipes:* When I transitioned to a vegetarian lifestyle, I was determined to adapt our family recipes while keeping their essence intact. I remember the first time I made **Kare-Kare** using peanut butter and a medley of vegetables. My daughters were skeptical at first, but as they took their first bites, their eyes lit up with delight. It reminded me that food is about experimentation and joy—an opportunity to create something new while honoring the past.

These personal stories are a testament to the role food plays in our lives, weaving together the threads of our culture, family, and love. As you dive into the recipes in this book, I hope you find inspiration not only in the flavors but also in the connections they foster. Let's celebrate the joy of cooking, the richness of our heritage, and the love that nourishes us all.

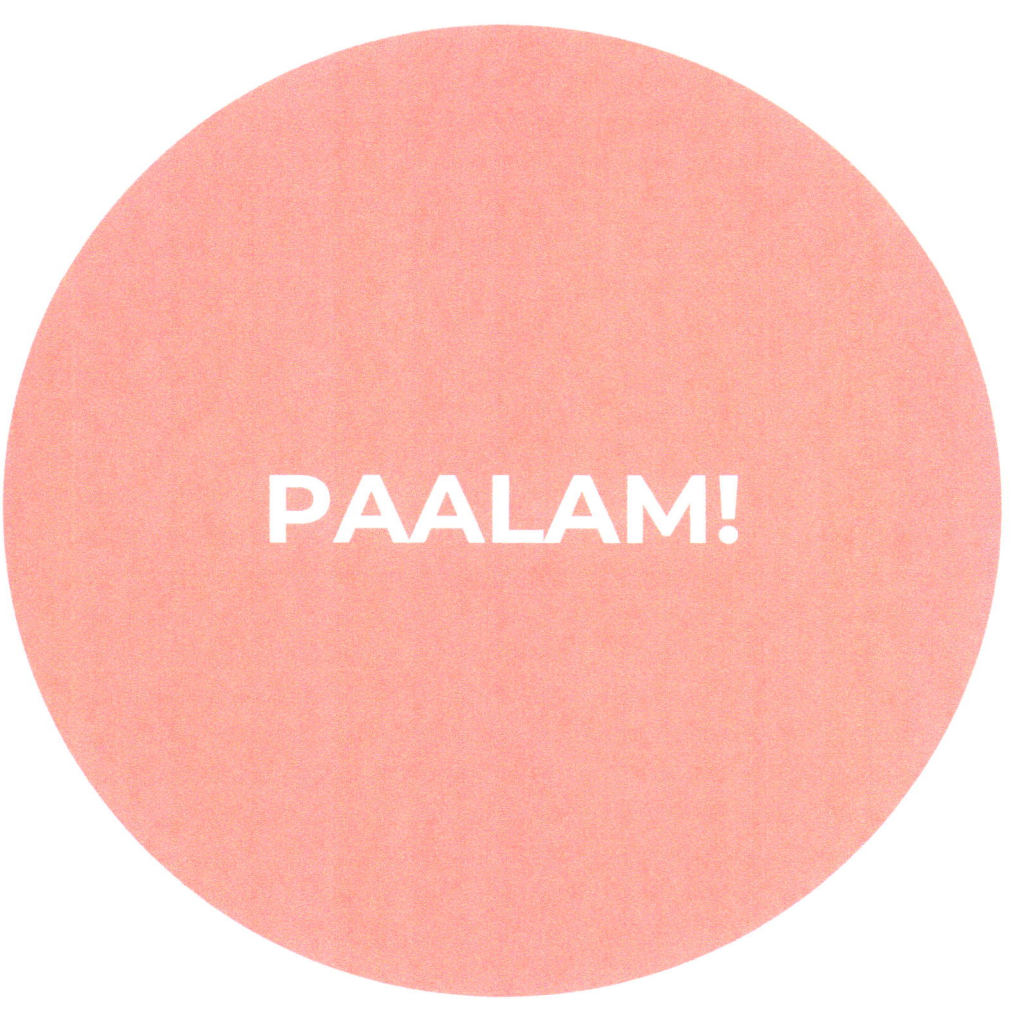

Celebrating Filipino Heritage Through Cooking

As we reach the end of this culinary journey together, I want to take a moment to reflect on the beautiful tapestry of flavors, traditions, and memories that Filipino cuisine brings to our lives. Cooking is not just about nourishing our bodies; it's about celebrating our culture, connecting with our roots, and sharing our stories with loved ones.

By embracing vegetarian cooking, we honor the rich culinary heritage of the Philippines while making choices that are kind to our bodies and our planet. Each recipe in this book is a tribute to the vibrant flavors of our homeland, reimagined to fit a plant-based lifestyle. Whether it's the comforting warmth of **Sinigang** or the indulgent sweetness of **Leche Flan**, these dishes are more than just food; they are a celebration of our identity, our history, and our shared experiences.

I encourage you to continue exploring the diverse world of Filipino vegetarian cuisine. Let the flavors and aromas inspire you to create your own memories and traditions in the kitchen. As you experiment with these recipes, remember that cooking is an art—there are no strict rules, only your creativity and passion. Don't be afraid to add your personal touch, try new ingredients, and share your culinary creations with others.

Thank You and Encouragement
for Your Culinary Journey

Thank you for joining me on this journey through **"Filipino Flavors Made Meatless."** I hope this book has inspired you to embrace the beauty of Filipino vegetarian cooking and has filled your kitchen with love, laughter, and delicious aromas. Your willingness to explore plant-based adaptations of cherished recipes speaks to your commitment to health, sustainability, and cultural appreciation.

As you embark on your culinary adventures, remember that the heart of Filipino cooking lies in the joy of sharing meals with family and friends. Each dish you prepare is an opportunity to connect, to celebrate, and to create lasting memories. Whether you're hosting a festive gathering or enjoying a quiet dinner at home, let the flavors of your heritage guide you.

Paalam! May your kitchen be filled with the warmth of family, the joy of cooking, and the rich flavors of Filipino cuisine. I can't wait to hear your stories and see how you make these recipes your own. Here's to many happy meals ahead!

With love and gratitude,

INDEX

www.ingramcontent.com/pod-product-compliance
Lightning Source LLC
Chambersburg PA
CBHW071716140626
46557CB00011B/730